The Poultry Farmer's and Manager's
VETERINARY HANDBOOK

Peter W Laing

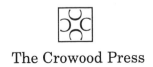

The Crowood Press

First published in 1999 by
The Crowood Press Ltd
Ramsbury, Marlborough
Wiltshire SN8 2HR

British Library Cataloguing-in-Publication Data
A catalogue record for this book is available from the British Library.

ISBN 1 86126 261 2

Acknowledgements

I have received help and encouragement from a large number of people during the preparation of this book and my thanks go to all of them.

Firstly I would like to thank the clients, especially Sir Simon Gourlay, David Styles, Russell Williams, Julie Burton and Ray Link, who allowed us to take photographs on their farms. This is coupled with thanks to Richard Stanton who took immense trouble with all the photographs that he took professionally and succeeded in making the filming sessions really good fun. Also thanks to Rosemary Morris and Claire Jones for their assistance with them.

Next, permission to use photographs and transparencies was generously given by Intervet UK Ltd., Bayer Pharmaceuticals, Maywick Gas Brooders, Harlow Bros. Poultry Houses, Kaycee Veterinary Products, the Department of Veterinary Pathology University of Liverpool, the Veterinary Laboratory Agency and the Central Veterinary Laboratory.

Finally particular thanks to Pat Owen and Anne Green for their endless patience and accuracy in typing, restructuring, retyping, altering and annoting the script, and to my wife Joan for help with the text and for putting up with me during the long gestation of the book.

Typeset by The Florence Group, Stoodleigh, Devon
Printed and bound by Redwood Books, Trowbridge

Contents

Foreword

Over the last fifty years poultry production has undergone considerable expansion throughout the world and this has been stimulated by the continuing increase in acceptance of poultry meat and eggs in the human diet. In many countries poultry production has become increasingly specialized and integrated into a dynamic industry. Simultaneously there has been an increase in intensive management and understanding of the significance of breed, housing, nutrition and preventive and therapeutic medicine to the health, welfare and optimal production of stock.

Disease and suboptimal production are of considerable economic importance to the poultry industry and it is now well appreciated that they are multifactorial in cause. Thus attention to all aspects of management is essential to minimize losses and it is of value to know how best to care for stock in health and when to seek specialist advice.

The Poultry Farmer's and Manager's Veterinary Handbook deals in a straightforward and comprehensive manner with the essential aspects of poultry keeping which are helpful to the beginner and also useful to the experienced farmer. It encompasses the poultry industry, the breeder flock, problems in hatching, management of the chick, broiler, roaster and egg production, normal and abnormal behaviour, and welfare. It provides an outline of the causes of disease, diseases of the systems of the body, immunity and the principles of resistance to infection, vaccination and treatment, and the value of hygiene in disease control.

There are a number of useful texts in all these subjects written by specialists for specialists but there is a need also for the manager and poultry keeper to have a general background on these subjects. The background should be a guide to the appreciation of health, suboptimal production and when it is necessary to request specialist help. This handbook provides such a background.

The author, a practising poultry veterinarian for many years, has written from his experience in the field with large flocks as in integrated groups and also the flock kept as a hobby. This book should be helpful to the farm manager or the amateur in maintaining health in a flock, in obtaining optimal production and also when to seek veterinary advice.

F.T.W. Jordan MBE, FRCVS, DSc, DPMP

Introduction

I hope that this book will help all those concerned in the management and health of poultry, whether of individual birds or large commercial flocks, to appreciate the fine balance between health and disease in chickens and to be able to establish the *reasons* for the various health problems so that effective treatment can be carried out.

There are a number of excellent textbooks and illustrated commercial publications written on poultry diseases and poultry health but the conditions are mainly described from the basis of the pathological lesions to be found at postmortem examination, from serological investigations and other laboratory tests. This book, written with my experience as a practising poultry veterinary surgeon over many years, attempts to provide a link with these text books by describing and discussing conditions as they are first seen by the stockman or vet on the farm. I hope that it will assist poultry keepers, whether large or small, whether poultry keeping is a hobby or a commercially run business, whether they are employed by one of the large integrations that make up the poultry industry, or are involved in chicken management in some other way, to be able to recognize and interpret the health problems that they encounter. They should then be able to assess their significance with more confidence and know better when to seek veterinary advice.

Poultry owners are often disappointed that veterinary books describe so few home remedies for diseases in their poultry, but even for a poultry veterinary surgeon at least three-quarters of the advice he gives on the disease problems referred to him in practice relates to disease management rather than simple treatment with drugs. A short chapter has been included in this book on first aid and the treatment of individual birds but specific treatment is usually the job of the Veterinary Surgeon.

The poultry industry is enormous and poultry provide a high proportion of the protein food – both as meat and eggs – for most of the world's population. In the industry one must understand that the individual bird is primarily a unit of production, designed by selective breeding to have a genetic potential for a specific commercial function – for example, egg production, rapid growth or the production of a carcass with a high percentage of breast muscle. It is no longer a natural bird and it requires special conditions of husbandry and management in order to remain healthy.

This book describes some of the mechanisms involved in maintaining the balance of health between the chicken and its environment. Only healthy birds are able to withstand the additional challenges that they are bound to meet on any modern poultry unit, whether large or small.

1 Keeping and Caring for Poultry

THE POULTRY INDUSTRY

Poultry and poultry products provide the major source of protein food for the majority of the world's population. In Britain alone over 600 million broiler chickens are produced each year and there are 35 million egg-producing birds in the country. The keeping of poultry must therefore be seen in this economic context; in commercial terms whether we like it or not the individual bird is primarily seen as a unit of production. Furthermore, many nations in the world still do not recognize the concept of bird welfare and are relatively unconcerned about the quality of life of the birds in their flocks. The minimum standards of housing and so on for the individual bird in the large and very intensive commercial flocks that comprise the major part of their poultry industry therefore vary widely. Because

Britain is part of the international trading community this fact is of profound economic significance to the industry.

In Britain and some other developed countries guidelines are increasingly being incorporated into welfare legislation but this is not the case in many other countries. Whatever the legislation, however, in the last resort it is the qualities of stockmanship, motivation, sensitivity to the living birds and knowledge of the individual poultryman, whether he is looking after only a few individuals or a million bird unit, that have the greatest influence over the welfare, in the true sense of the word, of the birds in his care.

Much of the mass market for poultry products is dominated by a small number of very large poultry integrations in the developed world. In Britain there has also always been a hard core of commercial poultry farmers who have remained independent. Now there is an increasing demand for quality food products of all

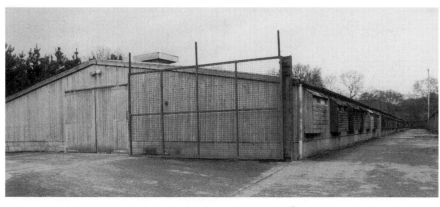

Fig. 1
A typical large broiler house with a security gate.

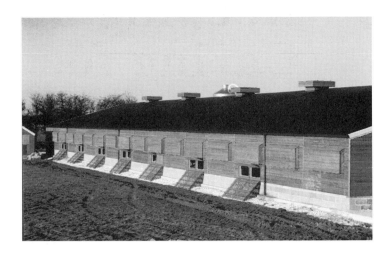

Fig. 2   A large free-range poultry farm.

kinds and both the catering industry and some supermarkets have recently started to look actively for producers of both poultry meat and eggs of a designated quality. This is leading to a welcome increase in the number of independent poultry producers running large poultry units.

Some poultry keepers maintain the Pure Breed fancy, and some families have been producing and showing their own birds for many years. Some of these flocks have poor health control, particularly if individual birds attend shows where they can pick up infection. A balance needs to be achieved between a hobby and a commercial enterprise and to remain suc-

cessful a disease-control policy for their birds is necessary and the birds that they sell must be free from disease. This is particularly important for those who sell pure-breed pullets commercially for the production of expensive quality eggs for niche markets.

Some poultry keepers simply like to have a few chickens pecking round the door and the birds are really companion animals like dogs or cats and have no true commercial function at all. Others like to keep a small flock to produce table birds or eggs for their own household. They get much satisfaction from keeping healthy stock of which they are proud, and in producing a good-quality natural food

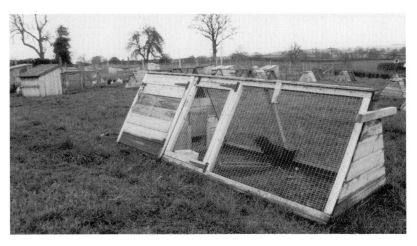

Fig. 3   A broody coop with run.

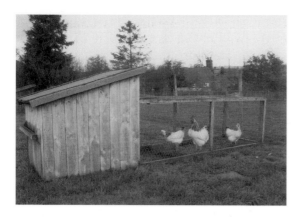

Fig. 4   A small-scale breeder poultry house.

product. For many of these people the experience gained leads them to start a commercial enterprise. This may start as a lucrative hobby, a diversification on a farm, or part of a catering concern.

Lastly some people drift into keeping chickens almost accidentally and this often leads to disappointment, misunderstanding and failure because unfortunately many of them do not fully appreciate the implications of keeping livestock.

STARTING A POULTRY UNIT

The implications of starting a poultry enterprise of any sort must be thought through in advance. The flock owner must decide whether:

- It is going to be just a hobby.
- It is a least-cost way of having a few living creatures around for the benefit of the family.
- Or it is to be a planned commercial poultry farm to generate profit.

Careful consideration should always be given to the possible health and disease risks. It is very important to build in a budget for both routine health care and veterinary supervision and for possible disease problems. If a poultry owner has not considered the possibility of running into an unexpected disease problem in a commercial flock there will probably be disappointment as well as expense because of failures in egg production, tablebird production or the quality of birds for sale. Sick chickens are unprofitable. They do not lay eggs or put on weight. Expert advice on health will be needed and the poultry vet should become a trusted member of the management team.

For small flocks the demarcation line between sentiment for an individual bird and commercial considerations must be carefully taken into account. The veterinary costs of diagnosing and giving advice on individual birds, of post-mortem and other laboratory examinations on birds that die, and on treatments and vaccinations are fundamentally similar to those that an owner of other types of domestic animal has to face. Unfortunately many small-scale poultry keepers do not appre-

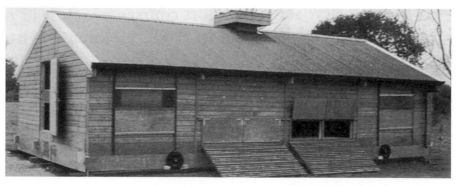

*Fig. 5
A Harlow free-range unit.*

ciate this and are horrified to find that they run up vets' bills as high as those that they accept as normal for the veterinary care of their dog or their daughter's pony. Small-scale poultry farmers must also realize that costs of vaccinating their chickens are heavily weighted against small flocks because the smallest vaccine pack available for some diseases is often for a thousand doses.

The next important point that must be considered before starting up any type of commercial poultry business is the requirement to comply with current legislation. Poultry are classed as food animals and are therefore subject to the legislation that relates to food safety. This means that producers, whether large or small, of any poultry product for sale must be able to show that they have taken adequate measures to ensure that any product is fit for human consumption, and that hatching eggs, chicks or pullets for sale are free from Salmonella. There are other requirements relating to welfare, slaughter and animal health and these are described later (Poultry Production and Human Health).

The health of the foundation stock taken over to start a poultry enterprise, however small, should be considered. Are the birds carrying disease? Are they infested with either internal or external parasites? Have they been vaccinated against the common locally occurring diseases or are they at risk from picking up infection from other birds already brought onto the farm?

There are a large number of very varied diseases that affect poultry and on long-established farms kept under traditional conditions, or in established collections of exotic poultry or pure-breed chickens, tolerance to many of these infections has been built up so that most of the birds remain clinically healthy most of the time. However, these birds are frequently carriers of diseases that have the poten-

tial to flare up if opportunity offers. If the birds are sold or transferred to start or add to another flock the stress of the change of management and location often leads to clinical disease a few days after the birds arrive at their new farm and this disease can then spread to other birds already on the farm.

Disease can also go the other way. If chickens already on the farm are themselves carrying infections they can pass these on to the introduced birds. When a new flock is started by acquiring foundation birds from a number of different sources at the same time the likelihood of disease breakdowns occurring is greatest and the possible routes of spread between the individual birds more complex.

Poultry keepers should have a basic understanding of all these factors when they start a new poultry enterprise and it is wise to discuss their proposed policy with their veterinary surgeon in advance.

POULTRY VETERINARY SERVICES

There are a small number of veterinary surgeons who specialize in poultry in general practice and these run practices that service all sectors of the poultry industry. The professional and technical service that can be offered is of a very high standard. The amount of information available to them from scientific sources all over the world is immense, for the poultry industry is a high capital industry with extensive technical back-up services. It should be appreciated that an average commercial broiler chicken farm in Britain consists of more than 100,000 birds. These are processed every seven weeks and therefore the average farm rears a million birds a year. Commercial egg-laying farms are also large and a farm with less than 5,000 birds is regarded as small.

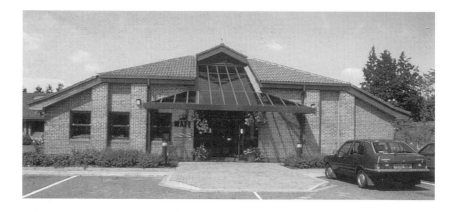

*Fig. 6
Bury St Edmunds
Veterinary
Investigation
Centre.*

These farms must therefore have comprehensive health and disease-control policies in order to remain profitable, and they require a highly efficient technical veterinary service. They need large budgets for preventive medicines, vaccines, farm hygiene products and veterinary services. Some of the biggest poultry integrations employ their own veterinary surgeons and in addition to these and the private practitioners there is a back-up service offered by the Veterinary Laboratory Agency. This service formerly called the Veterinary Investigation Service, used to be an integral part of the State Veterinary Service within the Ministry of Agriculture but, like so many other institutions, it has recently been partly privatized. The technical service they provide is available for all private veterinary surgeons and those who do not specialize in poultry usually use their technical expertise to help them make a diagnosis when dealing with a poultry problem for a client. Vets who do not specialize in poultry can also refer cases to poultry specialist practitioners. There is therefore no reason why every poultry farmer should not be able to receive expert advice on all his health and disease problems.

Specialist poultry practices also use the Veterinary Laboratory Agency and the State Veterinary Service for in-depth assistance and a close relationship between the two arms of the profession is an integral part of the service that the poultry practitioner can offer. Technical facilities now available include histology, serology and virus isolation. In the past few years great strides have been made in recognizing viruses directly under the electron microscope, but great technical skill is needed to select the right samples from the bird for examination at this high magnification, sometimes as much as 50,000 times. Even more recently genetic coding and DNA examinations are

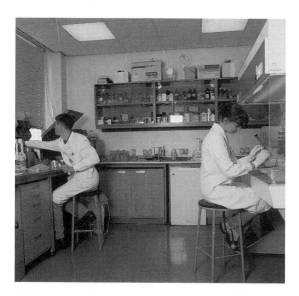

Fig. 7 A laboratory in a Veterinary Investigation Centre.

being developed to identify specific disease organisms and rapid progress is being made in this field.

Some poultry diseases are of such importance, either because of the devastating effect that they can have on the poultry industry itself or because the diseases they cause can be transferred to human beings, that they are under government control. The State Veterinary Service working with the Veterinary Investigation Service and practitioners operate these controls. Different countries in the developed world have legislative controls covering different diseases according to their regional significance. In Britain, Newcastle disease and avian influenza are both notifiable diseases. They are virus diseases that occur worldwide. Newcastle disease is potentially devastating to poultry, and influenza has additional public health risks because under some circumstances it can transfer to people.

Salmonella infections in poultry are also under some form of government control. One type, *Salmonella pullorum*, used to cause very high mortality in baby chicks from bacillary white diarrhoea and was controlled successfully by a state blood-testing scheme. Other salmonellae are those that can cause food poisoning in man. They are controlled by different legislation. The type most serious at present, *Salmonella enteritidis*, obtained instant notoriety in 1988 when Edwina Curry, a member of the British Government, stated that a high percentage (the majority!) of the eggs eaten every day in the country were infected. Other types of salmonella are also capable of causing human food poisoning.

The safety of poultry meat for human consumption is another aspect of poultry keeping that is under veterinary supervision. Controls have recently been brought together under the Meat Hygiene Service, a government agency, and all poultry

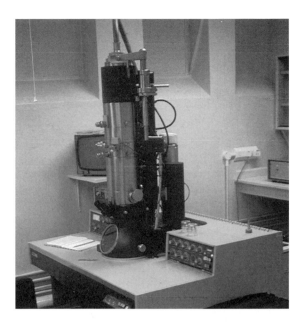

Fig. 8   An Electron Microscope.

owners who produce poultry meat for human consumption have to comply with this legislation. Official veterinary surgeons are appointed within the service to supervise all slaughter plants and ensure that the European legislation is being complied with, and the veterinary profession also has a central role in implementing poultry welfare requirements.

Every poultry farm that produces poultry meat for human consumption must now have a nominated veterinary surgeon with whom the OVS at the poultry processing plant can liaise if there is a problem relating to their slaughter. The nominated vet will be the farm's private vet. The poultry farmer must complete a simple flock report sheet with each consignment of birds for slaughter stating any disease sustained during growth and certifying that, if any drugs have been given, the required withdrawal periods have been complied with before the birds were sent for slaughter. The nominated vet's name will appear on this sheet and if the OVS has any problem with the birds

11

when they reach the slaughterhouse, either in the field of welfare, fitness for human consumption or compliance with medicines legislation he will liaise both with the nominated vet and the poultry farmer. From this it can be seen that the vet is an essential part of the farm's management team and gives help in the difficult business of complying with all the present legislation as well as being available to help to overcome health and disease problems on the farm.

Small-scale poultry producers are often surprised by both the scope of veterinary knowledge available to them and also by the legislative requirements with which they must comply. It is not always appreciated, although the evidence is there to see on our supermarket shelves, that poultry meat and egg products comprise a high percentage of the modern diet. Therefore, if infections in poultry that can cause disease in people are not fully controlled very severe outbreaks of food poisoning could often occur.

USING THE VET

A poultry vet will examine and give advice and treatment to individual chickens, whether they are pets, pure breeds or

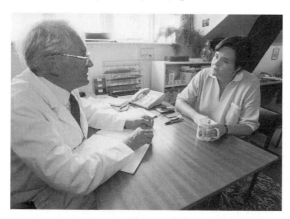

Fig. 9 *A consultation at the Veterinary Practice.*

members of a commercial flock. Usually, however, the advice required from him extends to the whole flock, whether it is large or small.

Major operations and complicated surgical and medical procedures can be carried out on chickens as on other animals but it is unusual for a poultry owner to consider that going to these lengths is justified. There are, however, vets who specialize in exotic avian species and rare breeds who undertake this type of work.

When a small-scale poultry owner consults his vet for the first time about the health of an individual chicken or a number of birds in his flock the first consultation usually takes place at the veterinary surgery. The poultry owner wants to know:

- What is wrong with the chicken.
- Whether it can be treated or will it die.
- Why it became ill.
- Whether people can get the disease from the chicken.
- Whether the disease will spread to other members of the flock.
- What action he should take.

Few diseases of poultry show absolutely characteristic symptoms in individual live birds. To come to a conclusive diagnosis on a problem that involves the flock and not just an individual bird, an in-depth investigation must usually be made probably requiring a post-mortem examination and other laboratory tests, whether the flock is large or small. This makes veterinary investigations expensive for a small flock and is a real problem for vets who undertake work for small poultry owners. Furthermore, the concept of destroying birds to establish an accurate diagnosis for a flock problem is one that many small flock owners find difficult to accept. Clearly the possibility of sacrificing a bird depends on the unit value of an individual bird; the flock may consist of valuable pure breeds of a rare genetic strain. In these cases 'blind' diagnosis without post-mortems will be the only option possible. Also some owners will not countenance destruction of any bird, and these must be treated individually as pets by the vet.

Another difficulty for small poultry farmers is that the poultry industry is geared for large flocks and the smallest packs of many vaccines and medicines available are for large numbers of birds.

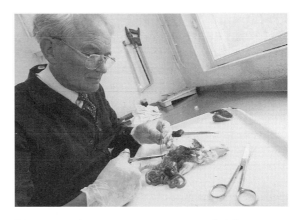

Fig. 10   A post-mortem on a chicken.

For a commercial poultry farmer, on the other hand, the vet should be an accepted member of the management team and it will be standard practice for the investigation of a disease problem to involve a partnership between an observant poultry stockman, the poultry vet and his back-up laboratory. Health problems are likely to relate not only to individual chickens but to the whole flock.

Laboratory diagnosis alone without a clinical and economic assessment of the problem on the farm is usually unsatis-

factory. In many cases several interacting factors contribute to a flock health problem. All of these need to be considered by the vet and the poultryman working together when deciding upon the best treatment and control measures to adopt.

When disease strikes a commercial flock it is normal practice to sacrifice a number of affected birds for diagnosis. If the disease outbreak is characterized by high mortality obviously birds that have died can be used for post-mortem diagnosis. However, most people working with

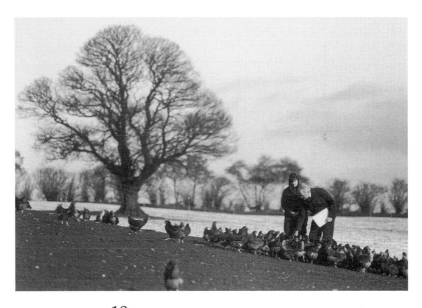

Fig. 11   A farm visit in winter.

13

poultry fail to recognize that death is really 'the end of the road' for disease and more is often learnt concerning the severity of the disease outbreak in the flock as a whole by examining living birds showing symptoms characteristic of the problem. Poultry health and disease problems are frequently multifactorial and veterinary advice can often involve recommendations on changes to management practices as well as treatment with medicines.

The poultry farmer's aim should be to categorize a health problem during his day's inspection of the flock and decide without delay if it is necessary to consult his vet or if it is purely a management fault that, having identified, he can put right. If he thinks that the problem could be food-related it is particularly important that he contacts the vet immediately and also that he takes a sample of the suspect food that the birds are actually eating (not from the bulk bins), and identifies this with the correct delivery date and ration code. If this is not done promptly and a serious problem develops and is found to be food-related it is often very difficult or impossible to prove liability of the feed company.

Similarly, if a health problem occurs within a few days of new birds, of whatever age, being purchased it is essential that the vet is notified immediately as well as the supplier. Then responsibility for the problem can be established if a legitimate claim against the suppliers of the stock or the transport company that delivered them is made.

Immediate treatment of a disease with drugs may be necessary on welfare grounds to relieve suffering in the birds, but the expense and long-term cost-effectiveness of the treatment and the effect of the disease on the future performance of the flock must also be considered. If it is an infection, a policy should be made to limit the spread of the disease to other flocks and to prevent its recurrence in the future.

Laboratory confirmation of a spot diagnosis made by the vet on the farm on clinical grounds is usually necessary in a commercial flock. It cannot be over-emphasized that accurate diagnosis is important so that future control and vaccination policies can be planned and the incorrect or unnecessary use of expensive vaccines and medicines avoided.

Some poultry farmers still think that vets are mainly drug salesmen and that their value relates solely to how cheaply they will supply medicines and vaccines. This is quite wrong. A conscientious vet will always be striving towards increasing the underlying health of his client's birds and making them less dependent on emergency medication. It may be that the price of some of the health products bought from him are a little higher than those charged by a retail salesman but this should always be weighed against the fact that the vet is not a *volume* salesman. He will be trying to help the poultry farmer to design an economic policy for overall health control based on the correct and most efficient use of the hygiene products, vaccines, parasiticides and preventive medicines available.

Food animals must increasingly be grown without the use of antibiotics or other additives. This means that all poultry owners need to get back to basics and have a real understanding of the different ways in which disease develops so that they are better able to keep their flocks healthy by more natural methods.

2 The Causes and Spread of Disease ─────────

THE CAUSES OF DISEASE

When the word 'disease' is mentioned most people think automatically of infection. This is always an oversimplification. There are factors other than infection that can cause disease in all animals and these are often very important in poultry.

Faults in nutrition can lead to specific diseases, and poisons and pollutants also frequently contribute to disease outbreaks both in intensive units and in flocks kept under more traditional management.

Environmental factors will cause disease or increase the severity of disease outbreaks from other causes. Poisonous gases may contaminate the air in the poultry house if the ventilation is wrong, and the temperature and humidity are also always important.

Often all the factors that can contribute to a disease outbreak are grouped together under the heading 'stress', and an understanding of what is actually meant by 'stress' is essential if poultry disease is to be understood.

All chickens, like human beings, are part of our biological world, within which they must achieve a balance with the ever-present disease challenges in their environment. René Dubos in *Mirage of Health* clearly writes how in animals there is a balance between health and disease factors and that this balance must always be maintained if the animal is to remain clinically in good health in its normal environment. This balance has particular significance with regard to poultry disease because of the widely varying environments and systems of management within which poultry are kept. These vary from the almost natural conditions for chickens kept in undeveloped rural countries or for backyard flocks in Europe, to the super-intensive controlled environments for cage-laying hens and broilers in the present-day poultry industry worldwide.

Critics of the extensive systems of management and of the philosophy of organic production state, quite correctly, that poultry kept under these management systems often carry more diseases than those kept in the very intensive systems that they wish to defend. Unfortunately, this is often true. The natural world is a biological world where every living species, whether it is a virus or bacterium, an intestinal parasite, or a bird or mammal, has evolved and survived by acquiring the ability to live in balance with the other living creatures in its environment. These may be predators, or organisms which in some way can parasitize it such as viruses, bacteria, or worms. If this delicate balance is broken down in a chicken the bird will become diseased but if the balance can be maintained infections can be carried without the birds showing any signs of disease. It is most important on an extensive unit that infections present in the flock, particularly any, like salmonellae, that are possibly transmissible to man are identified and the infections eliminated from the flocks. These 'environmental organisms' can occur in healthy chickens that show no obvious clinical signs of disease.

When larger and larger numbers of birds per unit area are kept together as a flock their environment becomes more contaminated, there is potentially more stressful competition between individual birds and the balance between health and disease breaks down. All the tools of poultry farming technology must be used to maintain the balance of health in poultry kept under present-day conditions. This applies equally to large free-range farms, pure-breed collections where birds are kept in small coops, or large commercial broiler farms.

If this balance is not achieved the birds live in a permanently stressful environment that will allow disease organisms already present in the environment of the farm to cause clinical disease. It will also make it easier for new disease organisms that are introduced onto the farm to infect the chickens and cause disease.

All poultry farmers should understand this fundamental concept of modern medicine. As a generalization, the larger the poultry flock the greater the degree of intensification and the higher the production targets for the individual birds (for example weight gain, egg production), the more dependent on 'good management' factors the birds will be if they are to remain healthy and profitable.

TYPES OF INFECTIOUS DISEASE ORGANISMS

It is now possible to consider the types of infectious disease organisms that occur in chickens and the ways that they spread.

Viruses

These infectious organisms are very small and can only be seen directly under an electron microscope with a magnification sometimes as great as 50,000. Even viruses are not the smallest organisms known that cause disease and the sinister virions associated with mad cow disease and scrapie are examples of these even more minute but deadly forms of life.

Viruses cause many of the most serious poultry diseases, for example Newcastle disease and infectious bronchitis, Mareks disease and Gumboro disease. The viruses live within the body cells of the chicken

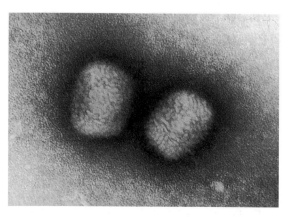

Fig. 12a   A pox virus.

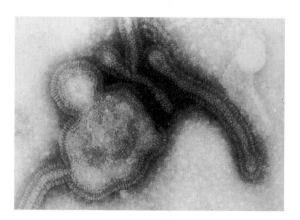

Fig. 12b   An ART virus.

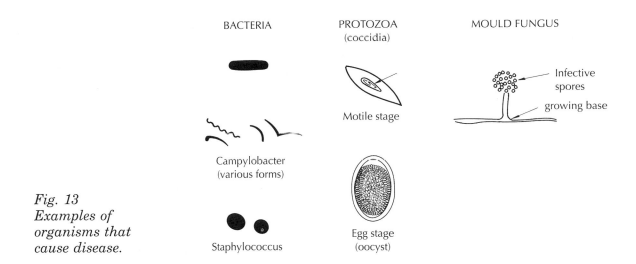

Fig. 13
Examples of
organisms that
cause disease.

where they cannot be readily killed by antibiotics. Many, like Gumboro disease virus, are also able to remain alive in a resistant form outside the chicken's body for over a year and some can take up residence in intermediate hosts like litter beetles and forage mites. When these are eaten by a chicken they can start to multiply and cause disease in the new bird. Some of the viruses that cause severe disease in chickens can also infect and multiply in other species of wild birds that can then spread infection from farm to farm. From this it can be seen that the complete elimination of some viruses from a poultry farm is very difficult and complete prevention of new infections occasionally reaching a poultry farm is not always possible.

Control measures must include:

- Reducing the disease challenge (number of viruses present) by good hygiene.
- Increasing the resistance of the chickens to clinical disease by good management and the reduction of stress.
- Vaccination against diseases that it is recognized cannot with certainty be eliminated from the environment

Bacteria

Bacteria are microscopic single-celled organisms and are present everywhere in vast numbers. Many species are useful and essential for the maintenance of life in all species, some are always harmful and cause disease and others, the facultative pathogens, can cause disease if the balance between health and disease in a chicken is broken down by stress or other factors, or if the bacteria are present in greater numbers than the bird can tolerate.

Before antibiotics became available it was the bacteria that produced primary diseases in their own right that were of most importance in poultry, for example cholera and bacillary white diarrhoea. Also, before the importance of hygiene was appreciated, environmental bacterial infections such as tuberculosis and staphylococcus caused very serious losses in many poultry flocks, and bacterial infections in developing eggs and baby chicks made the success of poultry breeding very uncertain.

Now in countries with developed poultry industries it is, in contrast, the organisms present in the environment that only cause disease under some circumstances that are of most importance.

These organisms, particularly the various strains of E. coli and salmonella, can cause disease in their own right if present in sufficient numbers but their ability to cause disease is vastly increased by stress factors or concurrent disease present in the birds. The study of the relationship between disease and stress is of great importance in the present-day poultry industry.

Fungi

Various moulds and yeasts can cause disease in poultry. The commonest is perhaps *Aspergillus fumigatus*. This mould is common in damp bedding, straw or fousty food and can cause severe disease in young chicks, either pneumonia or brain infection. Other fungi can infect the crop and other organs and some produce toxins that can contaminate poultry food and cause poisoning.

Protozoa

These are microscopic single-celled animals. They cause a number of serious diseases in poultry and are of great economic importance to the industry. The most important group in chickens cause coccidiosis. There are seven different species that can affect chickens and many more that cause disease in other birds and animals. They are more or less host specific; chicken coccidia do not affect farm animals and farm animals cannot infect chickens. This means that the answer to one of the questions commonly asked by poultry keepers, 'Can my birds pick up coccidiosis from sheep that have grazed the same field?' is 'No'.

Protozoa have a fantastic capacity for multiplication. Some, like coccidia, have very complicated life cycles involving asexual stages during which most of the multiplication takes place so that, for example, one coccidial organism swallowed by a chicken can produce over a million daughter organisms at the end of its life cycle of about five days, and each of these daughter organisms can infect a new chicken. This is why a disease outbreak from some types of coccidiosis spreads so quickly to all the birds in the flock.

Larger Parasites

The diseases caused by the more complex parasites such as worms are also classed as infections. A number of different species parasitize poultry and cause either digestive or respiratory disease. Some of these parasites, for example tapeworms, have very complex life cycles and in some bird species more exotic types of worm can infect the kidneys and other organs remote from the digestive system.

External Parasites

These are also important and can cause disease, poor production and irritability and behavioural changes in a flock. Lice are the commonest large external parasite; poultry keepers often believe their chickens have fleas but these are only very rarely found in Britain, it is lice that the poultryman has seen. Mites are very much smaller and resemble pinhead sized spiders, just visible to the naked eye.

THE WAYS DISEASE CAN SPREAD

From the descriptions of the different groups of organism that produce disease it can be seen that there are a number of possible ways in which the diseases they cause can spread. In fact in nature there are a vast number of different routes that are taken and these vary from simple physical contact to complex ones involving intermediate hosts.

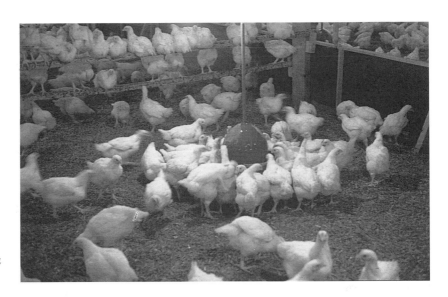

Fig. 14
Disease can spread via
the drinking water.

Spread by Direct Contact

Some external parasites spread by direct contact; for example lice and some species of mite. For the bacterial and virus infections that are caused by organisms so delicate that they cannot survive for long away from the bird, for example some respiratory viruses, it is the main method of spread. Of course many more resistant organisms can also spread in this way.

Spread in the Drinking Water

Delicate organisms, as well as many others, can spread quickly in the water that the birds drink. When a bird with a respiratory infection dips its beak into the water to drink, mucus containing large numbers of bacteria or viruses contaminates the water which can then infect the next birds that drink. Nipple drinking systems reduce this, but there can still be some spread from grossly infected birds. Stopping spread in the drinking water is particularly important for poultry-keepers in the control of fowl cholera or sinusitis.

If the original source of the water is contaminated, for example with droppings from pigs, calves or other livestock, or from overflow from farm effluent systems, infections can be transferred to the chickens drinking the water. Salmonella, other enteric disease and some parasites can transfer in this way.

Spread of infection within a poultry house often occurs when infected dust in the house settles onto the header tanks, drinking troughs or bell drinkers. All header tanks must have well fitting lids and troughs and bell drinkers must be regularly disinfected. Salmonella, E. coli, coccidiosis and some virus infections can all spread in this way.

Spread via the Droppings

In this method of spread the infective organism is passed out in the droppings. It may be immediately infective for another bird, for example in salmonella, E. coli and some viruses, or time may be needed for the organism to mature before it becomes infective, as is the case with coccidia and some other parasites. Infection is picked up by another bird either directly by pecking contaminated ground or indirectly by preening or by cleaning its feet when these have become contaminated.

When they have passed out in the droppings many of these infective organisms can go into a dormant stage and remain alive for very long periods. Many, such as Gumboro virus, tuberculosis bacilli, coccidea and roundworms can remain alive for over a year if environmental conditions are right for them. Some species have developed additional tricks that increase the possibility of their being consumed by another chicken. The large roundworm's (Ascaridia) egg, has a sticky shell that adheres to walls, plants, and therefore does not so easily get washed away out of reach of any new chickens to infect.

Spread in the Air

Infections can get into the air in a poultry house in many ways. In respiratory diseases they can be sneezed, coughed or breathed out. They can get into the dust in the air from dried droppings in the litter, from feather fluff and dandruff, or from infections that have been introduced into the house with vermin, wild birds and so on. Infections can also be introduced in dusty feed, in dust on transport lorries or visitors to the farm and their vehicles.

In the air disease organisms can be transported over considerable distances in currents of air in the poultry house itself, or over much greater distances in the wind.

If the weather is misty and there are water droplets present in the air these will attract small particles of dust that can contain disease organisms. These can then remain suspended in the air for much longer periods than in dry air. Several viruses can be transported in this way for distances of over twenty miles in some British winter conditions.

Poultrymen often do not realize how much air and dust movement there is in a poultry house. In houses ventilated by fans there is of course gross movement of air all the time. Apart from this, draughts are caused by opening and closing doors, currents are produced by the movement of the poultrymen around the house, and thermal currents develop round heating units. An additional important fact that a poultryman must remember is that air drawn out of a house through the outlet vents of one house can often be drawn in through the inlets of a neighbouring house and spread infection there very quickly.

In any infection in his flock that can be spread in the air the poultry keeper should assume that if one chicken in a house is infected all the chickens in that house, and probably all the birds on the site, have also had a chance to pick up the infection. Very large amounts of money are regularly wasted because this is not understood and initial treatment for a disease is limited to the birds immediately around the ones that first showed signs of infection.

Spread during the Clean Down

Even on farms where good hygiene measures are practised and there is a thorough clean down between every flock of birds in each house a serious loophole often exists that allows infections to spread. Farmers often disregard the inevitable blowing about of dust and dirt that is associated with the actual clean-down process and the movement of tractors, trailers and fork lifts. These movements spread infections to other houses still containing chickens and, even worse, reintroduce infection into houses that have already been cleaned. This means that new birds going into these houses pick up infection as soon as they are housed. If chicken litter or manure is badly stored or transported, or is spread onto fields to which other chickens or vermin have access, infections can often get back into other chicken flocks by this route. Hygiene on the farm is considered in detail later in Ch. 28.

Spread by People

Poultrymen can spread infection from house to house on their boots or working clothes, or in dust particles in their hair. They can also occasionally become infected themselves with poultry infections. They seldom become severely ill and usually do not know that they are carrying the infections but they can transfer them to their chickens. Examples are Newcastle disease and sinusitis. On farms with very poor hygiene facilities for the poultry staff, intestinal infections like salmonella can also be spread by poultrymen. This happens frequently in the less developed countries. Visitors to the farm also often introduce infection. This is an aspect of farm security that is difficult to control, particularly on farms that are open to the public and those with farm shops or other retail sales outlets and is also considered in Chapter 28.

Spread by Alternative Hosts

Sometimes disease organism can infect other species, from which the infection can get back into new chickens if occasion arises. There are two main groups of alternative hosts to consider in this very complex subject. The first are direct transport hosts that merely transfer the infection from one place to another. Infections like salmonella or cholera spread by rats and other vermin, or worm infections like Ascaridia spread by wild birds are examples. Some parasites that do not spend their whole life cycle on the chicken, such as red mites, can spread by being picked up by transport hosts such as sparrows that get into the building. Similarly infections that the sparrows carry can infect the chicken house.

Gumboro virus can survive after being eaten by an intermediate host, a forage mite or litter beetle, within which it can remain secure and has a good chance of being consumed by another chicken, in which case it can start infection in that bird. Some parasitic worms produce eggs that, after passing out in the droppings of infected birds, can be swallowed by earthworms or slugs which, when eaten by another chicken, infect that new bird.

The other type of spread by an alternative host is when the disease organism undergoes some further development in it before it becomes infective again for another chicken. Histomas, the protozoon that produces blackhead, and also tapeworms, are examples.

Many of the parasites that cause disease in chickens can themselves act as intermediate hosts for smaller disease-producing organisms. Nature has evolved a fantastic web of routes and possibilities whereby each species, whether it is a protozoon, a virus or a worm, can survive from generation to generation and retain its niche in the natural world.

By understanding these methods of natural survival of disease organisms poultry farmers, whether they have responsibility for a small or a large flock, can successfully plan a health-control programme for their birds and are also better able to control disease when it occurs.

Finally, just as weather patterns in a country change dramatically from year to year, so the prevalence of particular disease organisms may also change. Change also occurs within the diseases themselves, either by the emergence of new strains as has happened in recent years with infectious bronchitis, or by actual mutation in the organism itself, as is particularly common with influenza viruses. Evolution is a dynamic process and organisms can change, so that their virulence and ability to cause disease are subject to variation.

3 Management of Poultry Flocks and Baby Chicks

KEEPING A BREEDING FLOCK

Many pure-breed collections are open to the public, either for them to select birds that are for sale or as part of an exhibition. In any case the possibility of infections being introduced should be considered. In flocks where birds are taken to shows there is also always the risk of cross-infection. Birds can pick up infection from those in neighbouring cages and birds carrying infection without showing symptoms can infect other birds at the show. Contact is often very close and bacterial infections such as sinusitis (mycoplasma) are often transmitted as well as external parasites. In fact some of the more exotic parasitic conditions like scaly leg mite are seldom found except in exhibition birds.

Ideally, show birds should be fully vaccinated against the most common poultry diseases but there is a problem for owners of small flocks because most vaccines are only available in bulk packs for a minimum of 250 or 1,000 birds and are also not routinely stocked by the majority of veterinary practices. Advice should be obtained from a veterinary surgeon who specifically carries out poultry work or from a recognized pharmaceutical company.

Birds returning from show should be kept in isolation for two weeks before being reintroduced into their flock in case they have either picked up an infection at the show or the stress associated with showing brings on a latent respiratory infection. If this does happen the bird can spread this infection to the other birds in the flock with which it has been in contact.

When new blood is introduced by purchase of additional birds these should always be quarantined on arrival in case they are carrying infection. Advice on specific policy should be obtained from the vet but they should always be wormed and treated for external parasites. These birds are valuable to the farm and a blood test to check their health status may well be economically justified. A course of treatment against any mycoplasma infections that they may be carrying may also be recommended. If the flock that they are joining is vaccinated the vaccinations of the bought-in birds can be brought up to date during the time they are in quarantine.

The farm should also have a disease-control policy for the replacement birds that are reared from a day old and also for birds for sale. Pure-breed chickens are valuable and can command a much wider market if they can be sold with a certificate relating to their health and vaccination status.

Susceptibility to specific diseases varies between the individual pure breeds and particular blood lines within them. Some breeds are particularly susceptible to Mareks disease and a strict hygiene regime coupled with effective vaccination is essential if rearing and selling birds of these breeds is to be successful. Mortality may be as high as 80 per cent in badly infected flocks. The chicks can die at any age; during rearing, at point of lay just after they are sold, or when they are fully mature. Needless to say, purchasers become disappointed and dissatisfied and avoid buying any more birds from the breeder concerned.

On the other hand, some strains have a very high natural immunity to certain diseases and for many years some successful poultry breeders have selected strains to increase the natural resistance of their stock. Before effective vaccines were readily available disease control by genetic selection was more important than more recently and great progress was made in natural control of both leucosis and Mareks disease. Recently this type of positive control has become more important again and rapid progress is possible using DNA technology.

Some diseases are transmitted direct from the parent breeder to the fertile egg so that the developing chick is infected before it hatches. Mycoplasmas, that make all types of respiratory disease more severe if they are present, and certain types of salmonella are examples and need specific control measures.

On small hobby farms and pure-breed collections chicks are reared in small groups. A broody hen may be used to incubate the eggs and then look after the chicks in a coop with a small run, or the chicks may be hatched in an incubator and brooded under hot lamps or gas heaters. When a broody hen is used the risks of her spreading infections must be recognized. Mareks disease is a particular problem because the most efficient way that the virus spreads is in feather follicle dust and dandruff from the hen. Vaccination at day old, when it is most valuable to counteract early infection, is difficult

when a broody is used because the eggs usually hatch over a longer period than when artificially incubated.

Fungus infection is often present in small incubators on pure-breed farms that are badly managed. If day-old chicks are bought from these farms there may be high early mortality from brooder pneumonia.

Where a single brooder house contains a number of pens each with its own heating unit, cross-infection between the different pens easily occurs. Early virus infections transfer in dust particles in this way because air is shared throughout all the house. Spread of infection between pens in the droppings can be controlled to some extent if a disinfectant footbath is placed outside each pen to prevent spread on the poultryman's shoes. However, when rearing chicks an all-in all-out system is much better with individual brooder pens for each hatch of chicks. Then the chicks can be reared in isolation from other batches of birds from a day old. Moveable coops or huts that have an exercise area and can be dismantled, disinfected and put up again on clean ground before re-use are excellent.

REARING PULLETS FOR EGG PRODUCTION

The choice of breeds available for commercial egg production on a large scale is fairly limited. The various hybrids are well advertised in poultry journals and may be seen and discussed at trade fairs such as the annual British Pig and Poultry Fair held in May at the National Agricultural Centre. Temperament, suitability for range management, appearance, potential egg production and egg colour are among the important points on which to select a suitable breed. The chicks will be bought in at day old straight from the hatchery or dealer. They will be

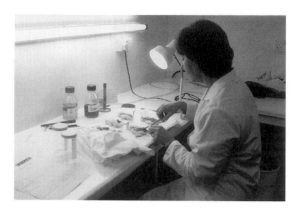

Fig. 15   Checking cause of disease in pullet chicks.

reared to point of lay at about eighteen weeks of age.

There is an increasing niche market for special types of eggs, for example the very dark Maran eggs and even the greenish ones produced by Aracaunas. For this market the day-old chicks will either be from parent breeders on the farm itself or will be bought in from other pure-breed collections.

The quality of the chicks at day old is obviously of great importance but their management during the first 24 hours after arrival, and then for the first few weeks of their life is also vital. This chapter later considers the management of baby chicks in detail. By the time a healthy flock is two weeks old there should be virtually no mortality or illthrift showing and it should be possible to begin to harden the birds off. After that age, when the birds no longer need constant heat, they may continue to be reared in the shed or, on more extensive systems, they may have access to paddocks. On large commercial units some pullets are reared in cages. Where pullets have access to range the exercising and grazing paddocks should not be continuously re-used by subsequent flocks; infections of all kinds will build up. The paddocks should be used sequentially and cultivated, prob-ably by ploughing and reseeding possibly coupled with grazing by sheep, before they are used again by chickens. The grass on paddocks for grazing must be fairly short and not too stemmy when birds first go out, otherwise impaction of the gizzard will occur.

Diseases and Vaccination

Pullets over two weeks old are suscepti-ble to coccidiosis and clinical disease will occur if the environment where the birds are kept allows the infective stage, the oocyst, to build up. At this age it is almost invariably caecal coccidiosis *E. tenella* that affects the bird. Vaccination gives excellent control of coccidiosis and re-moves the dependence on preventive med-ication using drugs.

When the pullets are between three and ten weeks old indications that a virus infection is present will show as mortal-ity and illthrift. The most likely causes are Gumboro disease or chicken anaemia virus but other diseases are possible and an accurate veterinary diagnosis should be made if a flock is not progressing satisfactorily during this period. Under conditions of poor hygiene when the level of environmental infection is very high the acute form of Mareks disease can also occur in pullets at this age, with mortality caused by rapid tumour forma-tion.

When pullets are reared in close prox-imity to older birds, respiratory infections are likely to spread to them, particularly after the pullets are a month old. Infectious bronchitis is the most common cause but Newcastle disease, turkey rhino-tracheitis and mycoplasma infec-tions should always be considered and, again, an accurate veterinary diagnosis made. If the flock is carrying *Mycoplasma synoviae* the birds may show not only respiratory disease during rearing but a severe lameness developing after the birds are about twelve weeks old. This is the classical form of the disease but has recently become less common. When it occurs it also affects the reproductive system of the developing pullets and flocks that have had the disease seldom become good egg producers. If mycoplasmal infection of any type is suspected an in-depth veterinary investigation should be carried out that includes all the birds on the poultry farm. This will include blood testing to detect carrier birds. The presence of these diseases reduces the possibility both of successful pullet rearing and of good production in the flocks reared and is disastrous for pullet rearers. Rigorous measures must be taken to control the infections.

As the pullets approach maturity, illthrift and death from Mareks disease may occur again in unvaccinated birds. This is very common in pure-breed flocks and on small farms. A post-mortem is necessary to confirm the diagnosis.

A vaccination and preventive medicine programme that includes control of all these conditions should be a part of good pullet management.

Approaching Maturity and Coming into Lay

When they begin to mature it is essential that pullets, whatever their breed, are well grown and big enough to sustain the stress of coming into lay. Otherwise reproductive disease may occur and egg production will be unsatisfactory. Also the number of hours of daylight that the pullets have during this phase of rearing must be controlled in order to delay the time that the birds start to lay until they are of the required weight for the particular management system to which they are going to be transferred. It is then essential for them to have extra hours of daylight to stimulate egg production. In nature the chicken, like the sheep, is a spring breeder and although selective breeding has developed the modern commercial hybrids into egg machines, the importance of a correct lighting pattern for them during rearing remains unchanged. It is useless rearing pullets in natural light during the summer so that they are just beginning to mature in August, when the hours of daylight are getting less. Failures to recognize the importance of increasing hours of light as a stimulus to production in point of lay birds is responsible for a lot of failures in small flocks. Healthy pullets that mature in August in flocks of this type often fail to come into production at all until the following February or March when the days are rapidly increasing in length again and the light intensity is becoming brighter. Also, if pullets fail to come into lay at the right age and become too fat during the winter their laying ability is greatly reduced.

Clearly, light control is impossible when pullets are reared on free range. For these poultry farms careful planning of the time of year that flocks are reared is therefore necessary.

Preventive Medication

Pullets reared for egg production will either be sold at point of lay or transferred to laying accommodation on the farm where they were reared. Consideration must be given to the system of management under which the chickens are going to be kept on the laying farm. Hygiene on many free-range farms is very poor and the young pullets will immediately be exposed to a very severe challenge from coccidia, E. coli and other disease-producing organisms. It is important that birds going on to this type of farm have developed a high level of resistance during rearing either by controlled exposure to infection or by vaccination. Veterinary advice on this important subject is necessary and the effectiveness of the vaccinations that the pullets have received must be checked before they are transferred. Failures to achieve a satisfactory immunity after vaccination are very common.

In all cases it is important that the pullets are as free as possible from diseases that they could transfer to the laying site and this includes parasites. This means that a strategic preventive medication should be given to the birds before transfer. A worm dose with a wide-acting anthelminthic can be given at this age because the birds are not producing eggs for human consumption. If worming is delayed until the birds are in lay, not only will they probably already have introduced infection onto the laying farm but also treatment may be uneconomical because eggs cannot be sold for human consumption until 14 or even 28 days after some drugs have been given in order to comply with medicines legislation. Treatment with insecticide against lice or mites can also be given at this stage. If the pullets are known to be carrying mycoplasma a course of treatment at this age will significantly reduce, but will not altogether eliminate, the number of carrier birds in the flock.

By the time the birds are transferred they should also have completed their vaccination programme so that their resistance to the diseases that they are likely to meet, particularly on multi-age laying farms, is at its maximum.

PRODUCING BROILERS, ROASTERS AND OTHER TABLE BIRDS

A successful producer of table birds must be able to supply his customers with quality carcasses passed as fit for human consumption in the right numbers, of the required weight, and at the right time. This is true whether the poultry farm is producing a specialized product for a niche market or commercial broiler chicken for a major purchaser.

In Britain over 80 per cent of the chickens grown for human consumption are either broilers or roasters and are grown intensively by the very small number of large poultry integrations that make up this part of the industry. A small number of genetic types of chick have been developed by the even smaller number of major breeding companies to supply this enormous market. These birds are very different from commercial egg producers and most of the pure breeds of chicken. They have a genetic potential for very quick growth, particularly of breast muscle, and are designed to be slaughtered at very specific ages that relate to their early management and nutrition. Broiler chickens are killed from thirty-six days of age and those kept as roasters will usually be slaughtered before they are eight weeks old.

To maintain the health of these birds in the very large numbers present on most broiler farms and produce carcases of good quality from them is a very skilled operation. The slightest faults in management, nutrition and disease control can result in a very high incidence of respiratory and bacterial disease, skeletal maldevelopment with lameness, and circulatory diseases. The welfare problems associated with these diseases are more serious because of the very large number of birds, often more than 30,000, that are kept in a single house.

Poultry meat producers, particularly those whose market is for quality birds outside the quite narrow specifications for which the intensive broiler breeds are designed, must maintain close control over the nutrition, environment and rate of growth of their birds. If they do not succeed in this they are likely to run into

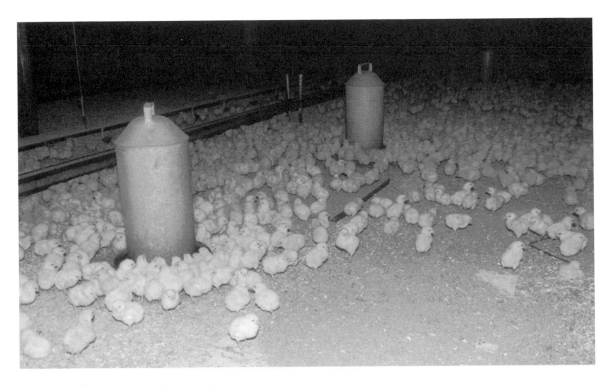

Fig. 16   Healthy broiler chicks.

high mortality from heart failure and dropsy, respiratory disease and skeletal developmental failures that will show as lameness, bone infections or gross deformity. If a flock of chickens being reared as table birds has any setback during development it usually remains a problem continuously; 'Once a jinx flock always a jinx flock' is a truism. Furthermore these flocks will usually produce an unacceptable percentage of carcasses that are rejected as unfit for human consumption at slaughter or are downgraded by the meat inspectors, increasing their unprofitability.

Whatever type of chicken is to be produced the chicks will almost invariably be bought as day-olds. Early management follows the same principles as for other types of poultry, but there are of course differences in nutrition. After a week, the later management of the birds will depend on the age at which they are planned to be slaughtered, on whether they will be reared indoors or on range, and also on whether they are to be reared within any constraints laid down by niche markets such as Organic Chicken, Freedom Foods, and so on.

The hybrids of chicken developed for meat production are very susceptible to Mareks disease. Usually vaccination at day old is needed. Poultry farmers who buy day-old chicks should find out from the supplier whether they have been vaccinated. If this has not been done vaccination on arrival at the farm is often good policy.

For birds that are to be kept on as roasters, especially those that will go out on range, a strong skeletal system is particularly important. Early exercise and the opportunity for the birds to develop their circulatory system is very important.

Broiler hybrids are docile and lazy and skill is needed to get the birds to exercise early in life, and to use their foot and toe muscles. Nutritional supplements containing additional calcium, phosphorus and vitamin D3 may be needed for birds kept on to heavy weights and advice should be sought when designing the feeding programme for the birds. If any lameness develops the vet should be contacted without delay because, in addition to the distress to the individual birds, lame birds do not grow well and do not produce top-grade carcasses.

If uneven growth or mortality are seen at any time the cause must be established and the diagnosis of any problems identified should be utilized in forward planning for the farm so that the same problems may be prevented in subsequent flocks being reared.

Respiratory diseases can affect birds at any age and are always serious and need to be positively identified. Often there are predisposing factors in the environment for the chickens. Sudden changes that result from birds going out on range, or being transferred to houses or open sheds that are not environmentally controlled, may all predispose birds both to respiratory and circulatory disease. Whatever the primary cause, disease makes birds more susceptible to E. coli infection and there will probably be deaths from E. coli septicaemia. Treatment with drugs may be necessary. Respiratory disease shows as sneezing or 'snicking' that is best heard in mild cases when the birds are at rest. There may be discharges from the eyes and beak.

It is normal practice for broiler chickens reared in sheds to receive medicated feed that includes a drug to prevent coccidiosis continuously. Birds going out onto free range and those reared under organic food systems where no drug is included in the food as a preventive are very susceptible to coccidiosis. For control they are dependent on good environmental conditions that allow them to steadily build up their own resistance or on early vaccination. The recently introduced vaccine is very effective and is proving to be of great benefit to poultry farmers.

If the litter in their house is poorly managed and wet, if the ventilation is poor so that there is condensation, or if the stocking density is too high in the shed or in the house when the birds come in at night off range, ulcerated feet (pododermatitis) and hockburn may develop. These conditions always indicate a welfare problem in the flock and also cause downgrading of carcasses at slaughter.

Grit is essential for the full development of the muscular gizzard. It is seldom given to broilers on intensive management that are killed before they are seven weeks old, but for birds that are to be transferred to range or barns with straw litter, grit is essential. The grit size should be as large as possible for the size of the bird and the stones should be sharp and not rounded so that maximum grinding can be achieved. In any case when birds are first transferred to range the grass should be short and not too stemmy, and straw bedding should not contain long strands of fine hay-grasses, or birds will get impacted gizzards.

Most meat strains of chicken are docile, but under some circumstances aggression can develop. Usually the cause is a management or environmental fault, or the presence of parasites on the birds or fomites in the litter which irritate the birds. Whatever the cause, as with any vices in chickens, pecking and aggressive behaviour quickly becomes a habit. It is, in any case, always good practice to give birds plenty to do, and suspending green vegetables and so on for them to peck at is good practice if there are any signs of aggression or boredom in a flock.

Whatever kind of table bird is being produced the conditions for carcass quality and food safety demanded by the customer must be strictly complied with. Chicken sold as organic under Soil Association rules must comply with their very strict rules and usually preventive medication is not allowed. Rules are also laid down by other purchasers, and supermarkets impose strict conditions on all their suppliers in order to improve the quality of the products they sell.

Birds on organic rations may sometimes need nutritional supplements unless the ration has been scientifically designed. Carcass quality is dependent on good nutrition and correct finishing of the bird before it is slaughtered. If the quality of the carcasses produced on the farm is poor, expert advice is always worth while. The problem may be disease, parasites, nutrition or faulty environment.

The health, quality and cleanliness of all chickens presented for slaughter is increasingly being checked to reduce the risk of human food poisoning and to verify that the chickens have been kept under satisfactory welfare conditions. Since the formation of the new Meat Hygiene Service these regulations are being applied to small on-farm slaughter houses as well as to the larger licensed poultry processing plants. Although compliance is irksome, the standards of many of these establishments was until recently quite appalling and regulations were badly needed both for the safety of the public and to check the welfare of the chickens processed there.

All poultry producers must have a clear understanding of the reasons for unsatisfactory growth, downgrading and carcass rejection at the slaughterhouse for any flock that they have produced. Chickens are classed as food animals and the health of the birds, carcass quality and food safety are all directly related. This means that there should be a close association between all poultry producers and their vets so that problems relating to health,

hygiene and welfare at any stage of growth of the flocks can be quickly investigated.

CHICK MANAGEMENT DURING THE FIRST FEW DAYS

On hatching, the baby chick's instinctive behaviour is to seek warmth, shelter and safety under the broody hen, and to explore in increasingly widening range in order to hunt for food and investigate its environment. Early exercise is vital for its development.

At first sight this may seem to be very different from the ways in which poultry are kept on commercial farms, but if a poultryman looks at a successful farm he will see that all these factors have been considered when designing the environment for the chicks, with one important exception. Many large commercial farms now use whole-house heating. In this system there are no separate heating units or natural mini-colonies of chicks within the house that may contain more than 30,000 birds, and there are basically no canopies under which the chicks can run if they are alarmed. Particularly skilled supervision is needed on these units because the chick's instinctive behaviour is not utilized in its early management.

Before a batch of day-old chicks arrives on the farm the whole brooder house must be heated to the correct temperature. It is particularly important to allow time for the floor and bedding to warm up so that the chicks do not chill when they settle down for their first sleep after delivery. The temperature must be maintained during the time the chicks are being housed. On badly managed farms it is often allowed to drop too low during this period and there are draughts within the house because the end doors are kept open.

Under traditional systems there should always be a gradient between the temperature under the brooders and the perimeter of the brooding area so that, if the chicks are marginally too hot, they can get away to a cooler part of the house. This also encourages the chicks to exercise and develop their muscles. However, the minimum temperature is also important otherwise there will be draughts in the house and the chicks will chill. Critical temperatures should be taken at the level of the chicks and checks should also be made at high points in the house and at places where it is thought there may be draughts. In this way an indication of the airflow through the house can be obtained as an aid in keeping the conditions in the house as constant as possible.

Guidelines for temperature control are that the temperature under the brooder should be between 90–95°F (32–35°C) and the minimum temperature at chick level should be 75°F (24°C). For a whole-house system the temperature is usually maintained at about 88°F, 32°C.

The quality of the air that the chicks breathe is also vitally important. Many poultry keepers still think that if the temperature is right everything else will automatically be right too. This is quite wrong and a significant percentage of veterinary problems investigated in practice relating to early mortality in chicks or their failure to get away to a good start are caused by the quality of the air that the birds have to breathe during those vital first days.

Gas burners burn oxygen and produce carbon dioxide and water vapour. Unless there are at least eight air changes per hour, reserves of oxygen in the air will fall and carbon dioxide will build up, together with water vapour.

If the ventilation in the house is very poor, the gas burners will not burn properly and will produce highly poisonous carbon monoxide. This will rapidly kill all the chicks under the brooder and is also an extreme hazard for the poultryman. Carbon monoxide is one of the most rapidly acting gas poisons and quickly causes sleepiness, headache, coma and death in anyone who breathes it. Carbon monoxide has no smell and accidents are common in the poultry industry. Irrespective of ventilation levels it is very important that gas burners are always adjusted correctly and are regularly maintained. The poultry keeper should never hesitate to contact the technical representative of the company supplying the gas burner if he has any doubts about the way it is burning.

It is very easy for a poultryman to monitor all these gas levels regularly by using a Draeger kit. Satisfactory levels are given in Ch. 9.

If the air is too humid the chick's lungs cannot function properly. They become congested and then fill with fluid, predisposing the birds to respiratory infections if they do not actually die. Conversely, on farms where electric or hot-air heating units are installed air can quickly become too dry. In this case the chicks overheat and die from dehydration and kidney failure. When dead ones are picked up they are sometimes quite crisp, like the roasted sparrows on sticks sold on market stalls in the Far East!

On delivery the day-old chicks should be of even size. Routinely weighing a random sample of delivered chicks before they are taken out of their boxes is a most useful management guide for all flocks. The chicks should be bright and active as soon as they are released from the boxes in which they were delivered. They should quickly be able to become familiar with their surroundings and find both the food and water provided for them. Chicks that cannot find food, particularly the weaker ones, will start to peck in reflex fashion

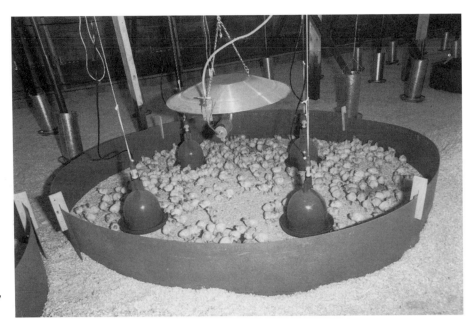

Fig. 17 A well-adjusted gas brooder and baby chicks.

at the bedding and will fill their stomachs with indigestible fibrous material so that there is no room for the chick crumbs even if the bird finally succeeds in finding the food. To help this it is important that there is a difference in colour between the crumbs and the corrugated paper or other material on which the first feed is spread. Some chick crumbs are not bright and refractile and even healthy chicks find them difficult to differentiate from the background material. A good poultryman should recognize this as a potential problem and not hesitate to discuss it with the feed mill. On small farms some poultry-men even mix a few of the 'hundreds and thousands' that are sold for cake decorations with the first couple of feeds to attract the birds to the right place. Moving the lights can also often help to solve the problem.

Once the chicks are delivered, spread of infection via the droppings should be kept as low as possible. Chicks should be prevented from roosting in or grossly contaminating the drinkers and feeders, and feeding them on the floor should be stopped as soon as the poultryman is sat-isfied that the birds are well settled.

The lights should be placed to encour-age the chicks to use the feeders and drinkers and careful selection of the colour and design of individual feeders and drin-kers, and the design of the chain feeder, are all important. On many poultry farms, both large and small, the chicks regu-larly sustain a severe setback when the change from floor feeding is made. Prob-lems can also arise with insensitively used nipple drinker watering systems for the birds.

If the chicks are bedded on hardwood sawdust or a commercial litter that has been disinfected before being spread this may occasionally cause a problem. The heat from the heater unit may vaporize any disinfectant remaining in the litter, or any fungicide or other agricultural chemical that has been added to the saw-dust. This can affect the chicks' breathing and irritate their eyes.

With experience a good poultryman should be able to decide after two or four hours whether a newly delivered flock is

31

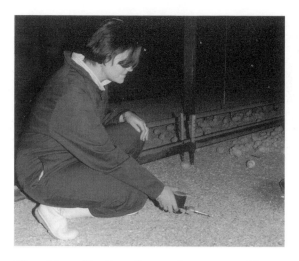

Fig. 18a   Testing for carbon monoxide using a Draeger Pump.

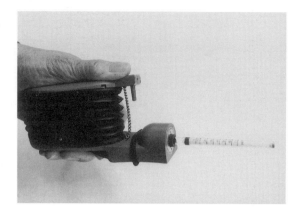

Fig. 18b   A Draeger Pump.

settling properly. If they are not, urgent action must be taken to establish the reason why. It cannot be stated too often that the first twenty-four hours after delivery are vital for the subsequent good progress of the flock being reared. A good poultryman looking after a traditional (and these are often unjustifiably maligned) poultry house will assess the environment for the chicks under his care from his personal experience. If they are too hot he will reduce the heat source and possibly increase the surrounding area so that the birds can get away further to cool themselves. If he thinks that the conditions for the chicks are stuffy or sweaty he will increase the ventilation by manually adjusting the windows or fan speeds. Faults in the environment provided for the baby chicks are very commonly encountered in veterinary practice, either if the poultryman is inexperienced or, often, if the environmental conditions are on a badly designed computer programme. There is a widespread view that computerization has been an unqualified advance in management but it cannot be overemphasized that computerized systems for regulating the environment for continu-

ously developing chickens are only as good as the computer programme. Unless a programme has been designed by a technical team truly experienced in rearing living birds under normal farm conditions it will be nothing like as comprehensive as that provided, hour by hour, by an experienced stockman who can modify the system instantly. Weather and housing conditions, particularly insulation, vary widely on different farms and in different countries and many computer programmes are very inflexible and rely on a very limited number of often badly placed sensors that measure only a very small number of parameters.

It is only if all the environment and management are known to be right that a poultryman can be sure that, if a problem occurs, it relates to the quality of the chicks, infection or early nutrition and not to a fault in his early management.

Developing chicks need light if they are to grow normally. Light induces activity and exercise and stimulates the birds to search for food and water. In some of the less docile hybrids for commercial egg production, and in some pure breeds, growing birds quickly develop aggressive behaviour

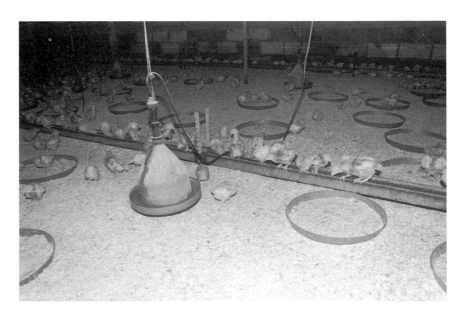

Fig. 19 Chicks spread infection when they roost on the feeders.

if the stocking density is too high, the colony size around the heater units too big, or if there are other faults in the environment. Many poultrymen reduce the lights to a very low level to counteract this. This is unsatisfactory because it reduces the level of activity in the flock to a stage where the food consumption falls and the birds cease to grow. Also, in windowed houses in summer attempts to reduce the light intensity by blocking up all the windows often lead to the ventilation in the house becoming inadequate with the resultant onset of respiratory disease or ammonia poisoning. In extreme cases where only red light is used to illuminate the house normal development of the chicks' eyes is prevented and they become blind.

EGG PRODUCTION

Successful independent egg-producing farms must plan their flocks so that they have eggs of the right size available for sale throughout the year. These day-to-day requirements will vary with seasonal factors such as tourism and demand from their major customers.

This means that unless the farm is part of a producer syndicate it is usually necessary to have more than one flock in production at the same time, which makes disease control much more difficult than on a one-age farm. There is a risk of introducing new infections onto the poultry farm with each point-of-lay flock that is bought in and also there is the probability that, when the new flock is introduced, the birds will pick up infections that are already present on the farm just at the time that they are at their most vulnerable and beginning to come into lay. On free-range farms some infections can contaminate the grazing areas and spread infections from flock to flock by this route. Intestinal infections including salmonella and some viruses are particular problems as well as internal parasites.

It is therefore important to maintain a vaccination policy, to buy vaccinated birds if possible and to check the health status of all the flocks on the farm periodically by blood testing at times advised by the vet. It is also wise to isolate newly purchased birds for a fortnight before mixing them with the existing flocks. During this time additional vaccines can be given. Also, if the start of egg production can be delayed by planning and careful management (and this planning will be influenced by the way the flock was reared before purchase), preventive treatment for external parasites, worms and coccidia can be carried out without the economic loss entailed in dosing birds during lay and having to withhold the eggs for sale because of the possibility of drug residues. If the chickens are bought from a farm known to be carrying one of the mycoplasmal infections, or in special cases where salmonella, E. coli or other bacterial infections have been a problem during rearing, antibiotic treatment may be advised by the vet during this period as a part of the farm's disease control programme.

There is no doubt that the disease risks on the very big one-age all-in all-out commercial egg-producing farms where the hens are all kept in cages can be less than on smaller multi-age farms where the chickens can be kept on more natural management systems. Useful lessons can be learnt by *all* poultry farmers by looking at the disease-control methods used on these giant farms on which there may be over a quarter of a million birds of the same age, producing enough eggs each day to feed all the people in a city the size of Leeds.

On these farms the birds are brought in from closely controlled pullet-rearing farms and are housed on an empty farm that has been prepared by a very rigorous hygiene disinfection programme. They have been vaccinated against all the diseases that it is thought likely they may meet during their laying life and the effectiveness of the vaccines given has been checked by a blood test before the pullets were transferred to the laying farm. A successful farm will also have a strict Unit Security Policy to reduce the likelihood of new infections being introduced with feed lorries, visitors, birds and vermin. Unless

there is a major epidemic of a virus infection such as Newcastle disease that can spread onto the unit in the air, the flock has a good chance of remaining disease-free during the whole of its laying life.

The risk of salmonella food poisoning is always in the news and assurance that eggs do not carry infection has been increasingly required by consumers since the 1980s. There is now a very effective vaccine against *Salmonella enteritidis*, the type that causes most cases of food poisoning, but control must also include strict hygiene measures on the farm and a realistic assessment of the particular risks that relate to it; for example from rats, birds or from a carry over of an infection from a previous flock. Good hygiene and rotational management of the grazing paddocks will reduce the levels of infection and regular monitoring of both the environment for the chickens and the chickens themselves by swab testing indicates whether infection with any species of salmonella is present and how widespread this infection is.

If salmonella is found, the laboratory that carried out the testing must notify MAFF under the Zoonosis Order. If there are good communications between the farmer, his private vet and MAFF, and salmonella control measures are seen to be a part of normal farm management, the draconian control by slaughter of the whole farm that made salmonella legislation so unpopular after the 1988 egg scare are not applied.

Complete eradication of salmonella is not always possible but it is increasingly becoming standard policy for all pullets going onto egg-production farms to be vaccinated against *Salmonella enteritidis* during rearing. The vaccine is expensive but is of great benefit to egg producers. It gives protection to the individual chickens, boosts the confidence of the farm's customers on the safety of their eggs and therefore increases quality sales and it

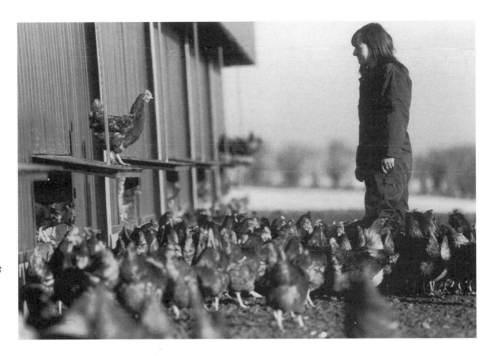

Fig. 20 Stones or weld mesh outside the pop holes keep the entrance clean.

also makes it easier for farmers to rid their farms of infection. An increasing number of supermarkets and other major purchasers of eggs are now requiring all the eggs that they purchase to be from vaccinated chickens and the British Lion Brand trademark can only be used if eggs come from farms that apply a salmonella control and vaccination policy. Unfortunately the vaccine does not give control against any of the other types of salmonella.

Disease challenges to birds in lay do not always show as clinical illness. A drop in egg production and an increase in poor quality eggs is always an indication that something is wrong and a sudden change in food or water consumption should also always be regarded with suspicion. Virus infections often have a particularly severe effect on internal egg quality whereas parasites and faults in nutrition tend only to influence egg size and shell colour.

Poultry farmers usually think of coccidiosis as a disease that only affects growing chickens. On free-range units, however, the litter in the house near to the popholes and also near to badly designed drinkers often gets wet and is an ideal site for the development of the infective stages. Pullets that have reached maturity without developing a good immunity to coccidiosis are often affected with clinical disease after egg production starts. The use of weld mesh or netting outside popholes so that the birds have drier feet when they enter the house, and also the replacement of the litter which is always wet with an area of netting or weldmesh inside each pophole so that the remainder of the litter can remain dry and 'work' effectively is often useful. Obviously, popholes should be protected from the direct entry of rain into the house. Any management practices that reduce the amount of contaminated mud entering a free-range poultry house on the birds' feet, and any other measures taken to reduce the amount of droppings that are consumed by the birds, either by direct pecking or by preening, will reduce possible levels of infections in a flock.

Gravel or road stone that drains quickly, can sometimes be used instead of weldmesh. All these factors are of great importance in disease control on free-range units, but are often overlooked by poultry farmers.

Individual management and separation of the grazing areas is important and rotational grazing of the paddocks should be practised. If the chickens can fly from their own paddock to another one containing birds from a different flock disease will easily spread. Control of wild birds is, of course, not completely possible and birds will unfortunately be attracted to the paddocks if feeding and watering the chickens on range is part of the farm policy.

In poorly ventilated houses birds will be predisposed to picking up respiratory disease and to a breakdown in their vaccinal immunity to diseases such as infectious bronchitis. In extreme cases the ammonia levels in a house can build up, particularly during the night, to levels high enough to cause ammonia poisoning and blindness.

In houses that are difficult to keep clean, particularly multi-deck percheries and houses with wooden nestboxes and inaccessible floor slats, red mite infections build up quickly. It is for this reason that a treatment against possible mite infestation is advised for pullets before they are housed, as this will reduce the number of carrier birds. However, infection can also be introduced by wild birds so absolute freedom from newly introduced infestation is not possible. Infection will persist in a house from flock to flock unless both maintenance of the building and thorough treatment with insecticide between flocks has been carried out.

Nutrition influences egg production and quality at all stages of production (see Chapter 9). The supply and type of calcium available for the laying birds is an important consideration because of the amount of calcium a laying bird needs to form each eggshell. An egg weighs about 2oz (60gm) and the shell contains approximately 2.2gm of calcium which has to be available each day when a hen is in full production. When calcium metabolism fails the hens can develop brittle bones (Osteoporosis). They suffer from many fractures and the egg shells become thin. In addition to extra calcium, provided in the right form, vitamin D3 supplementation is often very beneficial. These problems are much more severe in caged birds

Another indication of disease challenge in a flock is a sudden moult. One morning the poultry house is full of loose feathers and this may have started an outbreak of aggressive behaviour and feather pecking. Virus infection is often the reason, in chickens severely infested with external parasites feather loss takes place less suddenly. Any sudden change in the behaviour of a flock may be caused by an infectious disease and should always be investigated as a matter of urgency.

Legislation relating to the safety of eggs for human consumption is increasingly strict. A very real difficulty for all egg-producing farmers and their veterinary surgeons is that the medicines legislation to control drug residues in human food has made it increasingly difficult to treat birds for disease during lay effectively. When most drugs are used the eggs must be withheld from sale both during treatment and for a specified withdrawal period afterwards. This often makes the treatment financially disastrous for the flock because the withdrawal period may be for as long as 28 days after the treatment is completed. On the other hand, if the flock is not treated there will be an unacceptable welfare problem if the birds are obviously sick. In any case, in the absence of effective treatment egg production is likely to remain unsatisfactory

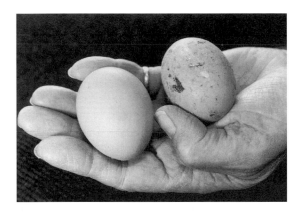

Fig. 21 Compare the good egg with the one laid on the floor which has picked up dirt.

and not return to a commercially profitable level.

Poultry flock owners must realize this fundamental problem relating to flock health and work closely with their veterinary consultant. With forward planning of vaccinations and strategic treatments before each flock comes into production the necessity for drug treatment during lay can be much reduced. In extreme circumstances the flock can be force-moulted and treatment and control measures taken before the flock is brought back into production. This sophisticated technique is often useful but must be carried out very skilfully. Technical help from ADAS and the poultry vet will be necessary for farmers carrying out the procedure and there are serious welfare considerations involved.

Dirty eggs and particularly eggs laid on the floor of a building are unsatisfactory for sale both because of their quality and

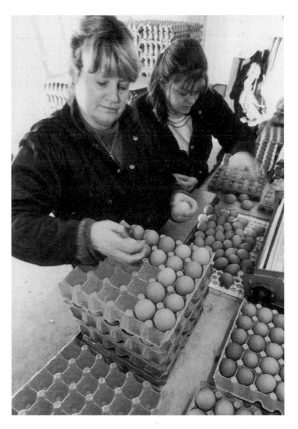

Fig. 22 Automatic egg collection on a moving belt is normal practice on large farms. The egg packers have to work fast.

because they can carry disease. Management of flocks as they come into lay and the design of poultry houses are important and advice should be sought on these points before starting an egg-producing farm. Eggs must always be collected frequently during the day and there should be no odd places in the houses where eggs can repeatedly be laid by birds determined to avoid the nesting boxes

4 Poultry Production and Human Health——

Poultry products are now the major source of animal protein in many countries. Because such large numbers of chicken are grown and eggs eaten any infections in them that can be transmitted to man and cause food poisoning are of great potential public health importance and a mass of legislation has built up to control this risk.

Infections in Chickens That Can Cause Disease in People

Salmonella
Most cases of food poisoning are caused by a small number of species of salmonella. These are not constant, but change over the years. At present *Salmonella enteritidis* and *Salmonella typhimurium*, particularly strain D104, cause most of the outbreaks in Britain. Salmonella can be present either in meat or in egg products.

Salmonella can infect anyone but the disease it produces is likely to be most severe in the very young, the old, and those with poor immunity to disease such as AIDS sufferers. People receiving certain types of medication are also particularly susceptible, for example those under treatment for allergies or asthma and people who have recently had organ transplants.

Campylobacter
This is another bacterium commonly associated with cases of human diarrhoea and enteritis. The organism is commonly present in chickens but does not cause significant disease in them.

Certain Types of E. coli
E. coli is a normal inhabitant of the digestive tract of all chickens, but some strains of the organism can cause disease in people.

Staphylococcus
This organism is present in very large numbers on dirty chickens and in skin wounds of all kinds. Cross-contamination at the slaughterhouse easily occurs and the infection can be transmitted to man, when it can cause severe food poisoning with vomiting and diarrhoea.

Other Infections
There are a number of other infections that chickens can carry that are transmissible to man but the diseases they produce are not common. They include avian tuberculosis and the fungus *Aspergillus*. The range of infections that cause disease is continuously liable to change, as happens in other food animals; BSE in beef is a good example. Conditions such as toxoplasma, virulent Newcastle disease and avian influenza can all cause disease. The recent crisis in Hong Kong, where avian influenza struck the chicken industry and was feared to be spreading to people, caused a public health crisis and is another example.

At the slaughterhouse carcasses can become contaminated with disease organisms either if the individual bird is infected or if the carcasses become infected by cross-contamination during processing. Unfortunately all of the infections cannot be recognized by the poultry meat inspector at the time the birds are slaughtered because most of the infected chickens remain as symptomless carriers. This means that effective control depends on rearing flocks that are completely free from disease organisms that can be transmissible to man. It also means that it is of the utmost importance to prevent any infection that does get into the slaughterhouse, whether it is a large poultry-processing plant or a small on-farm slaughter facility, from cross-contaminating other carcasses or poultry products.

Residues in Poultry Meat and Eggs

Another aspect of the Safety of Food for Human Consumption relates to chemical residues that can be present when the food is consumed. Governments are making progressive efforts to reduce and control the amounts of potentially harmful residues of all kinds that are present in foods, and the associated legislation has important effects on disease control in poultry.

The Meat Hygiene Service has developed over a number of years to tackle these problems. Each slaughterhouse is now supervised by an Official Veterinary Surgeon who is responsible both for the control of infections that can cause human disease and for the welfare of the poultry that arrive for processing. To help him to implement these responsibilities every poultry producer must complete a flock report form and send it to the slaughterhouse for each batch of chickens to be slaughtered. Each poultry farmer must have his own nominated veterinary surgeon who must be named on the form and who supervises the health and welfare of the chickens on the farm. Any illness that the birds have had during

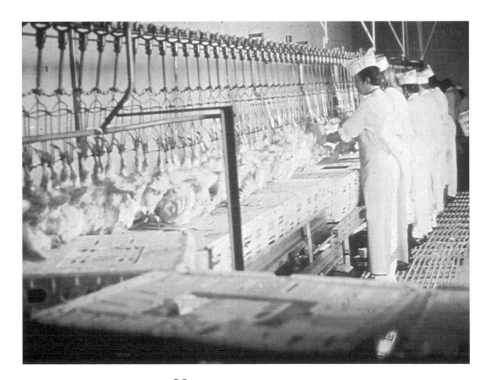

*Fig. 23
Poultry workers
in a broiler
processing
factory.*

39

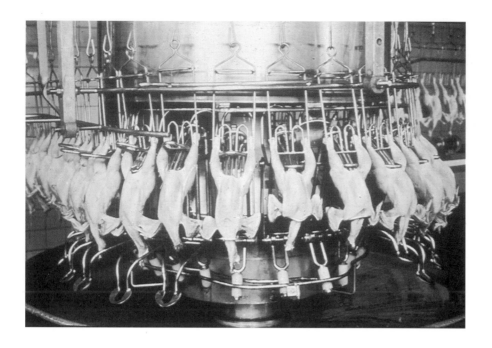

Fig. 24
Cross-
contamination
is inevitable
in a factory
preparing
broiler
chickens

rearing and any drugs that they have received, including in-feed additives, must be specified in the flock report. The purpose of this is to establish that the necessary withdrawal periods have been observed in order to ensure that no drug residues will be present in the carcasses at the time they are slaughtered, and also to give advanced notice to the OVS of any disease that may affect the carcasses.

To reduce contamination of the carcasses at the slaughterhouse with organisms that could cause disease, the Meat Hygiene Service attaches great importance to the condition of every batch of chickens when they arrive at the plant. It is important that the birds have not been fed right up to the time of slaughter. If the stomach and intestines are distended with food they easily rupture during evisceration and the contents spill out and contaminate the whole carcass and also spread to adjacent equipment. Salmonella and campylobacter readily spread in this way. Clearly, however, the poultry farmer must ensure that birds are

not deprived of food for too long before slaughter, the legal maximum being 12 hours.

Chickens that have been kept on wet litter or transported to the slaughterhouse in wet weather in open lorries arrive in a very dirty condition. Their carcasses are heavily contaminated and any infections they carry will spread to the equipment in the slaughterhouse and thus to other carcasses. The welfare of chickens arriving in this condition, or with sore feet or black hocks, has also been poor and there are regulations to deal with this aspect of the overall problem.

When the OVS sees a problem at the slaughterhouse that relates to the health and welfare of the birds on the farm he will contact both the poultry farmer and his nominated veterinary surgeon so that any necessary action can be taken. On a well-managed unit good use will be made of this liaison and a policy will be designed with the vet to improve the health and welfare of subsequent flocks to be reared.

Salmonella in Eggs

This type of infection is a very important potential source of food poisoning and is considered in detail in Ch. 13.

All poultry farmers should have a basic understanding of the infections that chickens can carry that can cause disease in people. Food Safety legislation makes it clear that if there is a complaint about the safety of any chicken product that was exposed for sale, or if a food poisoning outbreak is traced back to a particular farm, the poultry farmer must in law be able to prove that he practised 'due diligence' in producing the product. This includes a policy of Quality Assurance for the poultry products produced on the farm.

A Guide to Relevant Legislation

Food Hygiene General Regulations 1970, amended 1990

Poultry Meat Hygiene Regulations 1976

Code of Practice for Poultry Health Scheme Members 1988

Food Safety Act 1990, requiring registration of Farm Shops and so on in 1992

Poultry Breeding Flocks and Hatcheries Regulations 1989

Poultry Testing of Flocks Order 1989

Zoonosis Order 1989

Medicines Regulations 1994

5 Normal and Abnormal Behaviour

NORMAL BEHAVIOUR

Baby chicks in nature bond with the mother hen, and relate quickly to the group of chicks in the same clutch of eggs. They quickly relate to light and dark and initially associate darkness with security under the mother hen. Difference in the intensity of the light between the mother hen and her environment during daylight hours stimulates the chicks to explore, exercise themselves and search for food. This activity stimulates the circulatory system and the lungs and helps the birds to develop a strong musculo skeletal system from a very early age.

The external temperature greatly influences these activities. Chicks are very susceptible to chilling and under cold conditions in nature immediately return to the warmth under the broody hen, competing for the best position. If the chicks cannot get adequate warmth they very quickly chill. When chilled they keep up an incessant cheeping, stop pecking for food, become sluggish and die.

If the external temperature is too hot the chicks pant. They rapidly become dehydrated and can quickly die. They will also die quickly from respiratory failure if the humidity in the environment is too high.

As birds get older competitive behaviour becomes more marked. This varies widely between hybrids. Some are very docile, such as commercial broiler chickens and some pure breeds but others, particularly some strains of commercial egg producers, are much more aggressive. A natural pecking order develops within a flock of chickens of any age. The intensity of this again varies widely with the strain of bird. In nature it determines the maximum stocking density for the birds that are very territorial and compete for food, water and roosting places.

Poultry farmers should take the normal behaviour pattern of the birds into consideration when they are choosing a hybrid suitable for their particular farm. Aggressive strains of egg layers for example, although often very high egg producers, require a higher standard of stockmanship, better designed buildings and a lower stocking density than more docile breeds if problems from aggressive behaviour are to be prevented.

In breeding flocks, whether of pure breeds in small groups or pair mated, or in large commercial flocks, management of the breeding behaviour is important. In nature cocks compete with each other and the successful ones mate with a large number of hens if these are available. Unsuccessful ones are bullied, become stressed and may not continue to mate at all. If there are not enough hens for a cock (a ratio of about six to one is a fair guideline), or if pair breeding of pure breeds is being carried out, the cocks may overtread the hens and cause severe injury to them.

Hens coming into lay have quite specific requirements for their nesting sites

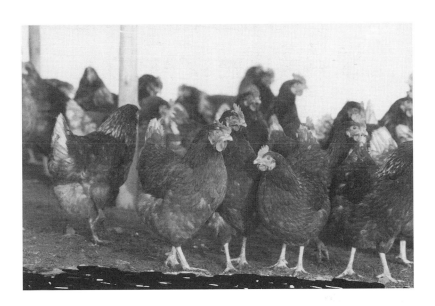

Fig. 25 A group of hens in a well-adjusted range flock.

and unless these are catered for in the design of the poultry house abnormal behaviour problems will quickly develop. A normal hen seeks privacy for egg laying and a fairly dark location. Slanting sunlight shining into a nesting box, or other bright lights, will deter her from using it. Ideally she needs to be undisturbed during lay and without competition from other hens. This is, of course, not possible when communal nest boxes are used. Easy access to the nesting box is particularly important and it must not be able to be obstructed or patrolled by dominant bully birds.

Natural competitive behaviour persists in every adult flock and mini colonies often develop within a poultry house where the stocking density and the house design is right and a comfortable balance has been reached between the dominant and submissive birds. In these cases groups of birds relate to particular feeders, drinkers, roosting places and nesting boxes. A good poultryman must remember this if it is necessary to catch up or move a flock for vaccination, anti-parasitic treatment of the house, or a change of location. Aggressive behaviour may be a

problem for a time after disturbance in a flock that was previously very contented.

Broodiness is natural at the end of lay for some breeds of chicken although it has been more or less completely bred out of the high egg-producing hybrids. When it does occur it may well be that there will be a demand for the hen from a smallholder for natural incubation of a clutch of eggs. Alternatively it may be necessary to remove the hen from the flock and break the broodiness. This is done by putting her on her own in an environment that in no way resembles a nest.

Pecking for food is another natural activity. This is clearly to be encouraged for birds on range, but on poultry farms where conditions are unhygienic and stocking densities high, parasites and enteric and virus infections can be picked up. This is a real problem in disease control on continuously used free-range paddocks and deep-litter units, in comparison with birds that are kept under fully controlled environment conditions on single-age sites.

Chickens actively appear to enjoy dust bathing and suitable dust bath areas should be incorporated into poultry houses when possible. This involves successful

43

litter management in the houses, otherwise on range units dust bathing will only be possible during dry weather, when the birds quickly make their own dust baths in suitable areas. Anti-parasitic preparations can sometimes be mixed into the dust baths to help to keep down the levels of external parasites in a flock.

The wild species of poultry from which domestic chickens have developed have many natural enemies. They evolved in-built behaviour patterns for their self-protection and these are still present in the modern bird. Instincts are to hide, or to fly or run away from a perceived danger and chickens are particularly aware of potential danger from above. This is clearly because hawks and other bird predators seek chicks and birds on the ground as their natural prey.

Some problems in chicken flocks where the birds are badly stressed are because farmers do not appreciate this. Panic situations in a flock develop instantly very easily. The birds attempt to run or fly away and can damage themselves or become smothered and crushed in very large numbers. It is most important that birds of all ages are kept so that they feel secure and do not panic when the poultryman, maintenance workers, or other people go through the flock. Birds should also be trained to accept sudden loud noises. Training the birds to feel secure is an essential part of good poultry stockmanship.

Normal behaviour patterns are part of the character of a species. All poultry farmers should be aware of the special characteristics of the chickens on their farm and allow for them in the environment and management of the flock. If this is not done the birds are likely to become excessively stressed and abnormal behaviour often starts. Behaviour such as egg laying away from the nests or wasting food makes a flock more difficult to manage and less profitable. Panicking, or any form of aggression quickly have much more serious consequences.

Poultry owners should understand the links between behaviour, stress and disease. Most so-called vices develop because of earlier management and environmental faults, or conditions in the birds themselves that have not been recognized. The poultry vet should always investigate in depth all aspects of the management of a flock that has developed a serious behavioural problem. Treatment confined to simple palliative or remedial measures alone without searching for the underlying precipitating factors will not enable the farm to prevent the same problem occurring in each successive flock. This happens very often in practice and is the reason why a lot of inexperienced poultry farmers give up altogether.

A certain amount of stress in their lives is, however, beneficial for any flock. In nature there is competition for a mate, competition for territory, competition for a high place in the pecking order of a flock and competition for food and water if this is short or if the stocking density is high. If a poultryman understands this he can appreciate that good management of his flock should provide the birds with enough stimulation to satisfy the requirements for the Five Basic Freedoms set out in the Welfare Codes. He should also be able to compare his management with, on the one hand, the stressful *negative* environment of some very intensive systems, and on the other hand with badly managed less intensive or extensive systems within which the birds are also subjected to excessive stress.

AGGRESSIVE BEHAVIOUR

Aggression and cannibalism can show up in a poultry flock of any age if there are predisposing stress factors. Problems are rare in the docile broiler breeds but very common in commercial egg-producing strains unless they have been specifically developed for docility, and in some pure breeds. The term cannibalism is used in a flock where the aggressive behaviour leads to the death of the attacked birds. It is the end-effect of uncontrolled aggressive behaviour in the flock and can develop from simple feather pecking very rapidly indeed.

Any alteration in the behaviour or appearance of individual birds in a flock can quickly upset the social equilibrium in the flock and lead to aggression. It is very important that a poultryman spots any changes in behaviour quickly as aggression is often the result of an earlier problem or a fault in the environment or management of a flock. Once an 'epidemic' of aggression develops, with severe vent and back pecking, sparring between birds and cannibalism, it is very difficult to break the bad habits that are remarkably quickly acquired by the birds. Drastic action is usually needed within hours rather than days and in an uncontrolled outbreak the whole social structure of the flock becomes completely disrupted and mortality may quickly reach 20 per cent. In a flock where aggressive behaviour is a serious problem there is always a significant number of subservient birds that become thin and go out of lay. They can be found skulking in the less obvious parts of the house and hiding under the equipment and machinery. These stressed birds usually die from kidney failure.

Feather Eating

The poultryman should distinguish between feather pecking, which is a sign of aggression, and voracious feather eating by a flock, when any loose feather is immediately gobbled up with great competition between birds, and the carcass of any bird that has died is eaten down to the skeleton within minutes of it dying. This behaviour will soon develop into aggression but its primary cause is often a nutritional deficiency. The birds are short of good quality protein that contains the amino acids necessary for feather development.

Predisposing Factors for Aggression

- Appearance of blood or abnormal colour on any of the birds.
- Poor feathers on the birds, leading to them having bare backs whose bright colour and exposed tail and vent attract other birds.
- Prolapse, abnormal exudate or caking of the vent.
- Too high stocking density for the house or the equipment in it.
- Poor design of the house, for example when bully birds can dominate key areas like the approaches to nests, feeders, drinkers, popholes.
- Number and design of feeders and drinkers. No bird should have to walk more than 3 metres to find food and water, and there should be easy access to the whole length of the feeders and drinkers for all the birds so that they cannot be bullied when they go to eat or drink.
- Incorrect siting, design and number of nest boxes. There should be one for every four birds except when communal nestboxes are installed.
- Competition for roosting spaces because of shortage of space, draughts or cold spots in the house.
- Bad lighting that allows shafts of sunlight to beam onto birds or equipment and stimulate pecking.
- Lack of facilities for normal behaviour so that the flock is bored. (No good litter, no dust baths, and so on.)
- Protein deficiency leading to feather and carcass eating that can soon develop into aggression.

- Loose feathers in a house when birds are moulting leading to competitive pecking.
- Irritation from parasites or vermin.
- Change of temperament in the flock due to disease. This is a very important predisposing factor, for example when birds have infectious bronchitis.
- Low salt in the ration.

CONTROL

- Pecked birds must be removed. They can be individually treated with a purple aerosol antibiotic spray advised by the vet and put in a hospital pen.
- The light intensity should be reduced and slanting sunlight eliminated.
- An attempt should be made to identify bully birds and remove them to a separate pen.
- Subservient birds should be found and moved to a separate pen.
- The environment should be diversified to reduce boredom. Vegetables and so forth should be suspended for the birds to peck at.
- Number, design and distribution of feeders and drinkers can be changed.
- Number of perches can be increased.
- Number of nesting boxes can be increased.
- Stocking density should be reduced if possible.
- Beaks can be trimmed on the advice of the vet.

Reintroducing birds that have been injured or bullied into the house at a later date must always be done carefully, preferably when it is dark and the birds are resting. The birds must be closely watched afterwards.

OTHER ABNORMAL BEHAVIOUR

It is always difficult to differentiate abnormal behaviour from illness. Signs of ill health are considered in detail in Ch. 6

Grossly abnormal behaviour indicates nerve damage usually from infection. Birds may stargaze, show tremors or convulsions, hold their heads permanently bent under their breasts, have their necks twisted in spasm or have an abnormal high-stepping gait.

Abnormal behaviour in baby chicks usually indicates illness or a serious fault in the environment. If a number of birds in a flock are showing nervous signs the possibility of Newcastle disease should always be considered and a veterinary investigation carried out. In most types of abnormal behaviour the condition is quickly copied by other birds in the flock.

Flightiness

Sometimes a flock shows a marked change of temperament and becomes very flighty, occasionally with simultaneous moulting and loss of feathers. If the change occurs suddenly it may be the result of infectious bronchitis infection. There are a number of other possible causes including nutritional faults, infestation with external parasites or parasitic worms, unsympathetic management, a change of stockman, the introduction of noisy machinery or workmen into the house, or fear of predators.

Head Shaking

A distinctive habit of head shaking sometimes starts quite suddenly in a flock of adult birds, often when they are around peak production. The whole flock is affected and if an individual bird is watched carefully it will be seen to momentarily stop what it is doing and shake its head rapidly from side to side, then resume its normal behaviour, to repeat the process periodically. The condition may be just a habit but it is often a sign of infection with one of the types of infectious bronchitis, in which case there will usually be a small but significant drop in egg production and quality. Sometimes an observant stockman can hear a slight but definite respiratory 'snick' if the flock is carefully examined when it is at rest. This provides a good example of how careful flock management and accurate record keeping can lead to a very mild outbreak of disease being identified. The diagnosis can be confirmed by a specific blood test.

Egg Eating

Eggs with weak or soft shells, eggs that break or crack after being laid or are stained with blood, all attract both the hen and other hens using the nest to peck at, and then eat them. This rapidly develops into a habit, when the hens consistently peck at normal eggs until they break, and then either eat them or carry them around the house. Eggs must be frequently collected during the day and any broken egg debris cleaned up. Roll-away nests prevent this particular problem to some extent. It may be just a habit, or due to bad lighting in the nest boxes but lack of calcium resulting in thin shells may be involved or infectious diseases that affect egg quality, for example Newcastle disease, infectious bronchitis or EDS (Egg Drop Syndrome). An investigation to establish the cause should therefore be made.

Vent Pecking

Any abnormality at the vent will attract both the bird itself and others that quickly notice it. Investigation from curiosity quickly develops into pecking, injury and then more pecking. As with anything that stimulates pecking, it can lead to unrelated aggressive behaviour. Individual birds with abnormal vents should be removed from the flock, and either treated or culled. If it is a flock problem the cause should be established.

Floor Eggs

When pullets or hens lay a large number of their eggs away from the nests the cause is normally a fault in some aspect of management, which may include failure to control aggressive behaviour in the flock.

Pullets must be trained to investigate and use the nests well before they start to come into lay. They should be discouraged from laying anywhere else by careful planning of the design and lighting of the house. Littered areas that are 'private' and badly lit will always attract birds to lay there. Even more importantly, the stockman must pick up any floor eggs several times during the day, if they are allowed to accumulate in any one place this will attract birds to lay there the next day.

If the number of floor eggs suddenly rises in an older flock it may indicate aggression or some other behavioural problem. If eggs are laid randomly about the building this may indicate infectious disease or fear and disturbance of the flock.

Wasting Feed

This is usually the result of using poorly designed feeding equipment, but boredom in the birds predisposes them to the habit. Beak trimming that has been badly carried out leaving the birds with a 'shovel beak' is also a predisposing factor.

Overtreading of Hens in Breeding Flocks

This is not really abnormal behaviour but indicates that management of the breeding flock is wrong. The ratio of hens to each cock or the space available in an individual breeding unit, for instance when pair mating in small coops, are factors that may be involved. Repeated or savage treading causes wounds on the back of the head often with infection and loss of feathers. Wounds from the spurs of the cocks can cause injuries to the body and flanks of the hen, particularly if she is poorly feathered. Removal of the spurs is classed as a mutilation and should only be carried out by a veterinary surgeon in exceptional circumstances.

Aggression in Cocks

Aggression in older cockerels both to the poultryman and to visitors, particularly in a pure-breed collection open to the public is a real problem. These birds are not suitable for retention.

6 Health, Ill-health and Stress ———————

SIGNS OF HEALTH

When they are written down the signs of health in chickens appear to be very obvious but in an everyday farm situation the variations from normal that may be present and may indicate a disease problem of some kind are often very slight and subtle. It is the early recognition of these signs by a good poultry keeper that is so important. It can lead to a quick call to the vet if he thinks it necessary, an early diagnosis of a problem, and the immediate start of treatment or other control measures.

The Daily Health Check

Most poultry flocks consist of a large number of birds so the daily health check must be designed on a flock basis; it is clearly not possible to handle each bird individually. However, the flock consists of a number of individual chickens and the poultryman must understand the signs of health or disease in the individual chickens in order to make an assessment of the health of the flock as a whole.

It is good practice for a stockman to go through a formal check list each day and record his findings, whether he is looking after a small or a large flock. These can then be kept with the other flock records.

The daily health check on the flock made by the poultryman should consist of:

- Mortality.
- Food and water consumption.
- Egg production.
- General appearance of the birds, their activity and behaviour.
- Uniformity of the flock.
- Character of the droppings and condition of the bedding/litter.
- Conditions noted in individual birds, system by system, respiratory, digestive, nervous, and so on.

If any deviation from the normal is found, a more detailed investigation of the flock should be made immediately.

Egg Production and Egg Quality

Recording these is an important part of the flock examination each day.

Food and Water Intake

These are important indicators of flock health. They should be consistent, and within the targets for the flock. In free-range flocks however, water intake is significantly influenced by weather conditions, and food intake will vary when birds are changed from one paddock to another.

The food and water consumption clearly varies with the age and type of chicken, also with management and the type of food given to it. The following tables serve therefore only as very rough guidelines.

Water and Food Consumption per Day

Chickens for Egg Production

Age	Water consumption per 100 birds		Food consumption per bird	
2wk	1gal	4.55*l*		
4wk	2gal	9.09*l*		
12wk	4gal	18.18*l*		
Adult hens	6gal	27.28*l*	100–130gm	3.53–4.6oz

Chickens for Tablebird Production

Age	Water consumption per 100 birds		Food consumption per bird	
1wk	1gal	4.55*l*		
4wk	2½gal	11.36*l*	65gm	2.3oz
6wk	3½gal	15.91*l*	100gm	3.53oz
8wk	4½gal	20.46*l*	130gm	4.6oz

General Appearance, Activity and Behaviour

Healthy chickens of any age should have a bright alert appearance when they are awake. The eyes should be wide open and actively looking around, there should be no discharge from the corners of the eyes and no puffiness or swelling either above or below them.

It must be remembered that baby chicks sleep very soundly between feeds when they are content. They sometimes lie partly on their sides and their eyes are tightly closed. Indeed, it is easy to get a real fright when quietly entering a brooder house and seeing the birds stretched out in large numbers! However, when disturbed, healthy chicks wake up instantly and resume their bright alert appearance.

Baby chicks that are contented are normally fairly quiet but very active. A high level of cheeping in the flock always indicates a problem particularly when coupled with uneven distribution across the house and huddling.

Birds in a flock of any age should be fairly evenly distributed through the house. On free-range sites good use should be being made of the range paddocks, making allowance of course for the weather and the time of day.

There should always be a fairly high level of activity in a flock and, in laying hens, a contented 'talking'. Hens in full lay that identify well with their stockman will 'squat' in front of him as he is walking through the flock.

Any signs of aggression or abnormal behaviour must be spotted. The birds must be given time to settle down to their normal behaviour during the routine flock inspection. If they are not, abnormal behaviour will probably cease and valuable clues will be missed. It is always important that birds are not disturbed by the presence of the poultrykeeper during inspections or other procedures.

Posture, Legs and Wings
- Birds of all ages should stand symmetrically and should not need to use their wing tips for balance. Lameness in one leg is obvious when a suspected bird is made to move. The toes should be reasonably straight and able to grip. There should be no swelling of the feet.
- There should be no twisting of the neck or other abnormal positioning of the head such as stargazing. There should be no abnormal pecking movements. These signs are all indicative of some kind of nerve damage and accurate diagnosis is necessary. Blindness in any of the birds should be spotted by the associated abnormal behaviour.
- The wings should be held symmetrically close to the body and should not droop. This can be an early indication of virus infection in chicks or Mareks disease in older birds.
- Baby chicks should not have spraddle legs and birds of all ages should find walking 'comfortable' and should not subside into a squatting position after a few steps. The feet should be clean and not crusted with caked droppings. The toes should be normal and there should be no swelling of any part of the foot.

Feathers and Plumage
- The baby chick should have bright fluffy down that should appear quite dry and not sweaty. There should be no caking at the vent.
- In older birds condition of the feathers can be misleading because of normal development and the replacement of down with feathers. However, the developing feathers should not appear dry and full of dandruff and there should be no broken feathers sticking out at right angles to the body (so-called helicopter feathers). These faults may indicate a failure in nutrition or a virus infection.

- Once developed, the feathers should normally be held flat against the body. Birds that stand with their feathers fluffed up are either cold or sick. Except in hens during a normal moult the feathers should not be loose. Loose feathers in the poultry house are often an indication of disease in the flock.

Beak
- A healthy beak should be straight and the upper and lower beak should meet symmetrically. If the beak has been trimmed there should be no swelling or exudate. At all ages the beak should be hard and bright and not scaly.

Comb and Wattles
- When present these should be brightly coloured and fleshy. Their size and basic colour varies according to the breed, whether the bird is in lay or, in a cockerel, sexually active, and also according to the weather conditions. A good poultryman will know what is normal for his flock at any time and will be able to spot any sudden or progressive changes.

Respiration
- Respiration should not be laboured, the beak should be closed and there should be no respiratory sounds. If the bird is overheated or fearful, respiration will be rapid with the beak open. If the nostrils are blocked with mucus or other exudate the bird will probably show 'pouch breathing' in which case the sinuses under the eyes swell slightly with each breath. This is always a warning sign of respiratory disease.

The Vent
- The healthy vent has a pale-coloured intact perimeter. There should be no scabs, sores, fissures, or evidence of bleeding or prolapse and no staining of the feathers around the vent.

51

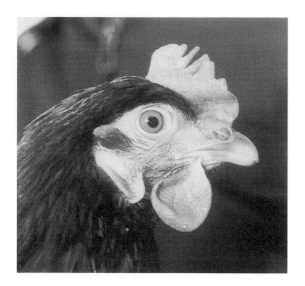

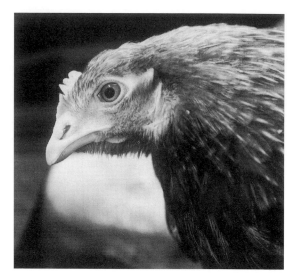

Fig. 26a   Well-developed comb of a hen in lay.

Fig. 26b   Shrunken comb of a hen that has gone out of lay.

Uniformity of Condition

In both laying birds and chickens for meat production uniformity in size and condition in the birds is an indicator of both health and production. A progressive unevenness in the birds can indicate a number of problems, many of them potentially very serious. Birds should be within their target weight for age. Confirmation of this will only be possible at regular flock weighings but a good poultryman should have a mental picture of how his flock should look and will spot developing faults quickly. Routine weighing of birds of all ages and all stages of production is an invaluable aid to good management of a flock.

Weight
● Birds should be within their target weight for age. Confirmation of this will only be possible at regular flock weighings, but a good poultryman should have a mental picture of how his flock should look and will spot developing faults quickly.

Droppings

A normal bird produces three different types of dropping.

1. Normal intestinal droppings which should be fairly firm and usually greyish brown, according to the diet.
2. Droppings from the caecum. These are a much brighter brown or orangey colour with a semi-solid sticky consistency.
3. Urine. The bird's normal urine is white and semi-solid. It is usually voided with the normal droppings and partly surrounds them with a whitish 'skin'.

The condition of the bedding (litter) and character of any individual droppings that can be seen at the flock inspection gives important clues to the health of the flock. The sudden appearance of wet litter is always serious. It may not only indicate diarrhoea in the flock but also severe kidney disease or a serious failure in the ventilation of the house. In all cases the cause must be established without delay.

SIGNS OF ILL HEALTH

The list that follows is not exhaustive but it is intended to give guidelines to a flock owner to help him to spot and interpret the signs in his birds that may indicate disease of some kind. The specific details of the various conditions are considered in the relevant chapters.

SIGNS OF ILL HEALTH IN BABY CHICKS

In chicks the signs of ill health in the individual birds overlap with abnormal behaviour shown by the whole batch of birds.

- Incessant cheeping and restlessness.
  Usually indicates chilling but can also be an early sign of disease.
- Huddling.
  Also indicates chilling, often from draughts.
- Chicks congregating round the perimeter of the brooder area.
  Indicates that the chicks are too hot.
- Chicks panting, often with spread wings.
  Chicks too hot, or poor air quality in the brooder house. For example, low oxygen, high carbon dioxide, high humidity.
- Chicks breathing rapidly, often with their beaks open.
  May also indicate that the chicks are too hot but is usually a sign of infection.
- Failure to find food and water.
  Probably indicates poor quality or weak chicks. May also be the result of poor management and environment for the chicks immediately after delivery, or of badly designed equipment.
- Chicks eating shaving, sawdust, and so forth.
  Indicates either failure to find food or early disease.

- Chicks standing alone with drooping wings.
  Usually indicates early infection.
- Chicks with swollen abdomens and prominent navels.

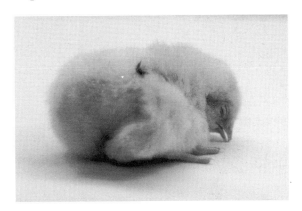

Fig. 27   A sick chick.

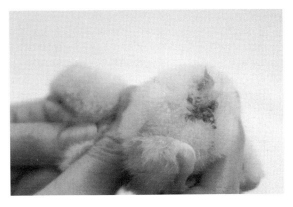

Fig. 28   A chick with a caked vent.

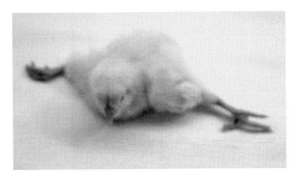

Fig. 29   A chick with spraddle legs.

53

Indicates yolk sac and navel infection.

- Chicks with caked vents.
  Indicates early enteritis.
- Chicks have spraddle legs and are unable to stand when delivered to the farm.
  Unless the chicks are being put onto a slippery surface on the farm this indicates a hatchery problem.
- Early aggression.
  Indicates environmental or management faults.
- Nervous signs.
  These usually indicate brain infection.

SIGNS OF ILL HEALTH IN OLDER BIRDS

Body Condition

- Thin or emaciated.
  May indicate chronic disease, lameness, stress, digestive disturbance, inability to eat.
- Obese.
  Excessive fatness affects the liver and reproductive function and may also cause prolapse or circulatory failure.

Posture and Distribution

Birds that stand, often on their own, with fluffed-up feathers are suffering from disease. If the whole flock is affected and huddled into groups it is either a severe flock infection or the birds are chilled. If birds are hiding under equipment this usually indicates aggression in the flock.

Lameness, Reluctance to Walk and Paralysis

Fracture, dislocation or swelling of one or more joints can usually be recognized by the poultryman, but in some other conditions the cause of lameness is not always easy to identify in a live bird, for example in hip lameness or paralysis.

If lameness is linked with any nervous signs the possibility of Newcastle disease must always be considered.

The great potential for very rapid growth and increase in body weight in broiler type breeds makes them very susceptible to locomotor problems of all kinds. Crooked toes and swollen feet should be noted. Conditions are described in Ch. 11.

Head, Comb and Wattles

The comb and wattles may be of abnormal colour. Deep purple may indicate circulatory failure or acute disease. Chalky white may indicate kidney disease. Scabs and ulcers may be the result of peck wounds, bacterial infection or pox. A shrunken comb in a laying hen indicates disease. A swollen head may indicate peck wounds that have become infected or a more general infection.

Beak and Mouth

Abnormality of the shape of the beak affects the ability to eat. If the beak has been trimmed, swelling at the base indicates infection. Nostrils blocked with exudate indicate respiratory disease. The mouth clogged with food may indicate specific disease, a food that is too pasty, or inability to swallow for some other reason. Scabs and ulcers in this region usually indicate infection.

Eyes

Closed, crusted eyelids, spasm of the muscles, blindness, exudate, opacity are all important indicators of a problem and are described in Ch. 17.

Neck

- Abnormal position.
  This indicates a disease of the nervous system.
- Loss of feathers.
  Particularly at the back of the head – may indicate feather pecking and aggression.
- Swelling at the front of the base of the neck.
  Indicates distention of the crop. When the swelling is squeezed sour food may be regurgitated (see Ch. 13).

Plumage and Feathers

- Bird standing fluffed-up.
  Indicates disease or chilling.
- Broken feathers sticking out from the body (so-called helicopter feathers).
  Indicates virus infection.
- Feathers dull in colour.
  Indicates disease.
- Feathers dry, possibly dusty or scaly.
  Indicates disease or a nutritional fault.
- Loose feathers or false moult.
  Indicates disease.
- Loss of feathers.
  This may indicate overheating, or particularly in laying hens, a sudden infection.
- Ragged plumage.
  This often indicates infestation with external parasites.
- Feather pecking.
  This usually indicates aggression but may indicate a fault in nutrition, particularly with protein deficiency.
- Staining round the vent.
  This indicates digestive or urinary disease or abnormality in the reproductive system. White staining indicates a urinary problem and brown or bloody staining indicates a digestive or reproductive disease.

Vent

- Caked with droppings.
  Digestive, urinary or reproductive disease.
- Sore and scabby.
  Infection from an unhygienic house or pecking wounds.
- Prolapse.
  Disease of the reproductive tract.
- Haemorrhage.
  Pecking or disease of the reproductive tract.

If any abnormality is present in a number of birds the cause should be established as a matter of urgency as the condition is likely to lead to aggression. Individually affected birds must be treated or destroyed on welfare grounds.

Swollen Abdomen

Birds show swollen tense abdomens, sometimes without feathers and with the skin a brighter pink than normal, because of congestion of the blood vessels. In birds of any age this may indicate circulatory failure and dropsy, or occasionally internal haemorrhage. In adult birds the cause is often egg peritonitis or, less frequently, cancer. The poultryman must be careful to differentiate any of these conditions from gross obesity. In all cases a post-mortem examination will establish the cause which may either be of flock significance or be a condition that only affects individual birds.

General Weakness and Collapse

This is seen mainly in adult hens or cocks. An affected bird is usually pale and unable to walk more than a few steps before subsiding to the ground. The cause is usually either heart failure or sudden haemorrhage. Haemorrhage may be internal or may be from severe pecking injuries usually involving the vent. Some affected cockerels are found in a collapsed condition with dark purple combs. These birds have had a heart attack and some will slowly recover if they are put on their own and individually cared for.

Care must be taken by the poultryman not to confuse general weakness with severe lameness or paralysis.

Respiration

Abnormalities are fairly easy to recognize but patience is needed when examining a flock so that its behaviour is normal and the flock is not still disturbed by the presence of the poultryman.

- Sneezing, gurgling breathing, gasping.
  These all indicate disease. The sounds are often slight and if in doubt of the presence of a respiratory condition the poultryman should visit the flock at night when the lights are out and the birds asleep. He will then be able to detect slight respiratory sounds if he listens carefully. Whenever a respiratory condition is suspected an accurate diagnosis is necessary because of the probably serious implications for the flock.
- Head shaking.
  This may be merely an acquired habit but it may indicate upper respiratory infection.
- Pouch breathing.
  This always indicates infection with obstruction of the nostrils and nasal chambers.
- Rapid breathing.
  This is always serious, it can indicate disease or overheating.
- Breathing with open beak.
  This again indicates infection or overheating and also possibly fear.
- Discharge from the nostrils or the corners of the eye.
  Usually indicates infection but may be a sign of ammonia poisoning.

- Swelling under the eyes.
  This indicates sinusitus and is an infection.

Droppings

First the type of dropping must be established, are they intestinal, caecal, urinary, or an abnormal discharge from the reproductive tract. An accurate assessment of any abnormal droppings is very valuable in establishing an accurate diagnosis of many diseases and is described in Ch. 13.

Nervous Signs and Abnormal Behaviour

Brain damage shows as some change in the birds' behaviour. They may show neck twisting or stargazing or the head may be held bent right under the bird's breast. Birds may make unnatural pecking movements and may not be able to find food. They may show an abnormal high-stepping gait or a change of temperament. For example the flock may suddenly become very flighty. Severely affected birds may have convulsions or tremors or become completely paralysed.

If a nervous disease is suspected the flock should be inspected quietly during the day. If birds are disturbed, nervous abnormalities in those that are only mildly affected will disapear and only the more seriously affected birds will show obvious signs. Where nervous disease is suspected the possibility of Newcastle disease must always be considered.

- Localized nerve damage
  This will show as paralysis of the affected area, for example, drooping of a wing, lameness or abnormal carriage of the head. Damage to nerves can lead to partial or complete paralysis.

56

Diseases of the nervous system are described in Ch. 16.

STRESS

The word stress is used frequently in relation to the health and management of chickens and indeed often appears in the text of this book. Everyone thinks that they know what stress is but it is nevertheless not easy to put its meaning into words.

Stress can be defined as a factor affecting the chicken's environment, management or physical condition that is unsuitable or disadvantageous for it. Stress can either cause illness and death directly, for example from kidney failure or can predispose the bird to abnormal behaviour or disease that it would otherwise be able to resist.

In flocks, whether large or small, in which there is not a good standard of management or a satisfactory balance between health and disease, problems are likely to occur that are in some ways stress-related and, in present-day poultry practice more than half of a veterinary surgeon's time is often spent investigating problems of this kind. There is clearly an overlap between stress conditions and those relating to bird welfare, which is considered in more detail in Ch. 7.

To assist in identifying any stress factors that relate to a particular flock the following areas should be looked at individually:

The Birds

- Breed, age.
- Stocking density.
- Colony size.
- Production.
- Quality of plumage.
- Behaviour.
- Beak trimming or other mutilations.

- Presence of disease or parasites.
  Disease of any kind in a flock always involves stress to affected birds and may also cause a change in behaviour. Sick birds are often bullied by the fit ones.
- Recent vaccinations
  Vaccination causes stress. For vaccine given by injection the birds must be caught up and individually handled. This must be done in a way that causes the least possible disturbance to the individual bird and to the flock. However it is done, the mini-colonies that develop naturally in a chicken house will be broken up during catching and there will be a period after the birds have been vaccinated during which stress-related problems can occur. By planning ahead most injections should be able to be given at times when a flock is being moved from one house to another as part of its normal management.

  In whatever way the vaccine is administered, live vaccines cause a different type of stress. Here the stress or vaccine reaction is actually the period during which the birds are suffering from the type of disease that is present in the vaccine. During this time the birds are under stress in the same way as they would be if they were suffering from a real disease. A special diet, vitamin supplementation, or even in some cases, specific medication may be advised.

Housing

- Structure.
- Equipment.

Environment

- Ventilation.
- Air quality.
- Temperature.

- Lighting.
- Condition of litter or grazing areas.
- Presence of predators.
- Presence of vermin.

Management

- Compliance with the Five Freedoms.
- Nutrition and availability of food.
- Any recent changes in management.
- Overall standard.

Whatever the system of management, the comfort for the birds depends greatly on the skill of the poultryman. Agricultural technology and scientific knowledge of disease have increased greatly since the intensification of poultry production began shortly after 1950. However, since then there has very often been a real loss of the empathy between the stockman and his birds that was once normal in farming.

7   Bird Welfare

Welfare means different things to different people and even the various definitions in different dictionaries cover a wide range of interpretations. The word has been overused in food animals in recent years and sometimes has acquired an unfortunate meaning, identifying bird welfare with over-regulation and interference in farming practice.

It is obvious that an outbreak of infectious disease immediately reduces the welfare of the birds or flock and taking a wider view, ill health for any reason is one of the most important factors that reduce a flock's welfare. Health and welfare are therefore the joint responsibilities of the poultry owner and the veterinary profession and in developed countries these responsibilities are incorporated into legislation.

Poultry farmers should understand the difference between bird welfare and frank cruelty. Cruelty is fairly easy to define and can be identified with actively callous or malicious treatment of the birds, or with gross neglect of any kind. Welfare, on the other hand, identifies more closely with the concept of the quality of life for the birds. Both cruelty and failures in bird welfare cause stress and in addition to the direct results of bad management stress-related conditions will develop. Stress upsets the balance of immunity of a flock to diseases such as coccidiosis, and the birds' susceptibility to infectious diseases of all kinds is increased. There are also a number of specific conditions affecting the health of a flock that have special welfare implications.

Concern for the welfare of poultry that did not relate to frank cruelty and neglect or infectious disease did not become an issue until the beginning of the intensification of the poultry industry in the early 1950s. From that time there was an increasing realization that there were serious adverse factors associated with over-intensification. These were related to what came to be described as the quality of life, whether for chickens kept in battery cages or large broiler sheds, or for pigs, veal calves or other domesticated food animals.

In Britain *Animal Machines* was written by Ruth Harrison and published in 1964, but scientists such as Professor Sydney Jennings, from the British Veterinary Association, sounded a note of caution in pointing out that the degree of discomfort or mental agony experienced by animals could only be assessed *subjectively* by human beings and that the boundaries between sentient and non-perceptive behaviour in domestic animals and birds were still ill-defined. A committee was set up under Professor Brambell and in 1965 reported on the implications of over-intensification. As a result of this, Codes of Practice for the welfare of animals kept under the various different intensive systems were progressively developed in Britain and implemented by legislation. The Codes of Practice for keeping chickens are clearly

59

based on 'The Five Freedoms' and these have also been incorporated into various marketing designations for poultry products. The Freedom Food trademark recently developed with much success by the RSPCA, and the older Organic Foods designation developed by the Soil Association are examples.

The Five Freedoms, as defined by the Farm Animal Welfare Council in Britain in 1992 are:

- Freedom from hunger and thirst.
- Freedom from discomfort (this includes the provision of shelter).
- Freedom from pain, injury or disease (veterinary supervision is a specific requirement).
- Freedom to carry out normal behaviour (this includes company).
- Freedom from fear and distress (this includes transport and slaughter).

Adoption of the Codes of Practice has led the British government to recommend a policy for a progressive reduction and ultimate ban on the keeping of chickens in battery cages. At one time over 90 per cent of the laying hens in Britain were kept in cages but the change in policy and positive direction given to the industry on welfare grounds has led to a progressive increase in the percentage of hens kept on so-called 'alternative systems'. The methods are actually, of course, the more traditional ways of keeping chickens, modified by the use of present-day agricultural technology. These more extensive systems of management have made great progress towards becoming disease-free and commercially competitive and supermarkets and other major purchasers of eggs are now buying these eggs in very large numbers and selling them under Quality designations.

Britain has always been in the forefront of matters relating to the welfare of animals and the ongoing 'Great Welfare Debate' involves the philosophical concept of the quality of life for all domesticated species, not only chickens, and the balance between purely economic factors and their freedom to exhibit normal behaviour that should be attained. Opinions go from the extremes of the Animal Rights movement, who think it cruel to keep laying hens for commercial egg production in the absence of a cockerel, to advocates of the battery cage system on the grounds that within the confines of the cage the chicken is safeguarded from exposure to many diseases.

When deciding which type of management system to adopt for their farm all poultry farmers must be clear in their minds on a fundamental point. Is the individual bird to be regarded solely as a unit of production in the same way as a ball-bearing or a plastic bottle on a production line in a factory or is each bird, however big the farm, to be regarded as an individual sentient member of a flock?

Two generations of people have now grown up since intensive systems for poultry became standard commercial practice and many of them have had little contact with farm animals in their urban community. When they are employed as stockmen it is very important that they both understand fully the difference between a living animal and a mere unit of production and conversely have a realistic approach to the necessity for a poultry farm to be profitable under the economic circumstances that apply at any one time. A poultry farmer must consider marketing possibilities and the commercial pressures that his unit will be subject to, not only from competition in Britain but from other countries both in and outside Europe. Not only is their attitude to bird welfare often very different, but labour costs, availability of land, cost of disposal of waste materials and freedom from legislative restraints all influence the degree of intensification possible and therefore the costs of production.

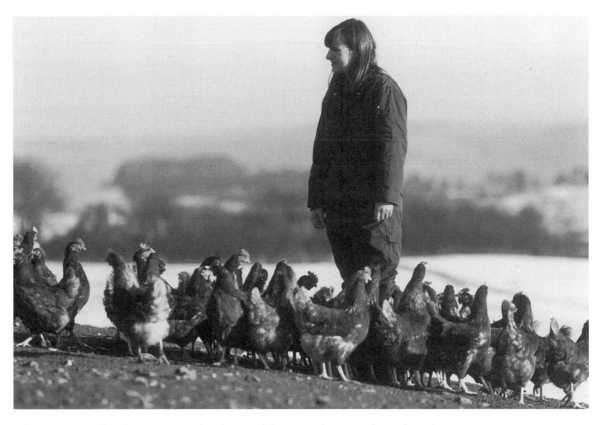

Fig. 30 The birds are completely confident with a good poultry keeper.

A poultry farmer must have an understanding of all these sometimes conflicting factors before selecting a suitable system of management for his unit, but real empathy between the poultryman and the birds under his care is by far the most important factor that contributes to the success of a unit, whatever the system. The degree of job satisfaction that all employees have is also vital in developing this empathy. The concept of welfare is a human one and not merely based on scientific facts and legislation. Control of health in a poultry flock is not possible without the full co-operation of the poultryman who looks after the birds. This simple fact has often not been recognized by companies that have adopted intensive systems of which their staff secretly disapprove. This has often led to economic failure of the farm and the development of serious welfare and disease problems in it.

Whatever system of management is decided upon its implementation must include:

- Proper planning.
- Caring management with adequate supervision of the birds. There should be at least two inspections by the poultryman each day.
- Satisfactory environment for the birds.
- Satisfactory arrangements for both table birds and hens at the end of their life for transport to the slaughterhouse or for actual slaughter on the farm.
- A policy for disease control and veterinary supervision.

There are, of course, many factors that relate to the welfare or quality of life of individual birds and these are discussed in various sections of this book and are listed in full in the various welfare guides for the management of chickens. Some specific points that are included in these welfare guides include:

- There should be no mutilations.
- The birds should have facilities for dust bathing.
- Green vegetables should be provided for the birds if possible.
- Birds on range should have access to shade.
- There should be no growth promoters in the feed.
- Slaughter of the birds should always be under OVS supervision.
- There should be a veterinary health and inspection policy for the farm.
- There should be variation in the height and location of feeders and drinkers in order to allow for differences in the size and temperament of the individual birds in a house.
- There should be a restriction on the maximum size of a flock.
- Separate pens should be provided for sick or injured birds.

Any disease or ill health affects the welfare of individual birds but there are some conditions that are clear indicators of a problem relating to the welfare, in the widest sense of the word, of the flock as a whole. A good poultryman should always be on the look out for the first signs of problems of this kind so that he can take action for the benefit of the birds under his care. Specific conditions include:

- Excess ammonia in the air
  This will lead to respiratory distress, irritation of the eyes and blindness. There is clear evidence of pain and discomfort in affected birds and the presence of the condition indicates a serious fault in the environment for the birds.

  Ammonia may build up because of a ventilation failure or overstocking. The legal maximum amount of ammonia in a workroom is 5 parts per million. A poultryman can usually detect that the level of ammonia in a poultry house is unacceptable when it reaches about 25ppm. There can be some clinical poisoning in chickens when the level is 50ppm but the gas settles into layers and in an affected house amounts measured in different parts of the house at different times of the day will vary widely and may be anywhere between 20 and 300 ppm in a problem house.
- Feather loss.
  This makes birds susceptible to chilling and aggression from other birds.
- Rapid change in the environment of a house after birds are thinned.
  This can lead to chilling and huddling. Care must be taken to maintain satisfactory ventilation and temperature control over this period.
- Poor cage design.
  Cages at best provide a very restricted environment for the birds. There are also still cages in use that do not allow birds to stand up straight and have steeply sloping floors and roofs. Cages of this type are illegal and cruel and must under no circumstances be used.
- Aggression in a flock.
  Remedial action must be taken as a matter of urgency. Injured birds must be removed and the underlying reason for the aggressive behaviour discovered.
- Lameness.
  Lameness is a complex problem in the hybrids developed for meat production. Their continually increasing genetic potential for rapid growth has led to a predisposition to a number of postural problems that present a serious welfare problem in many flocks. The frequent

STOCKING DENSITIES

(Different rates apply to different designations of hen)

Laying Hens

Traditional extensive system	max. 200 per hectare
Free Range	max. 1,000 per hectare + max. 7 birds/sq metre available floor space in the house
Strawyards	max. 10kg bird-weight/sq metre (guideline 3 birds per sq metre)
Percheries, single deck	max. 30kg bird-weight/sq metre (guideline 10 birds/sq metre) + Minimum percentage of 33.33% littered floor.
Percheries, multi-deck	max. 15.5 birds/sq metre + Minimum percentage of 50% littered floor

Batteries		
	1 bird in cage	minimum 1,000sq cm
	2 birds in cage	minimum 750sq cm per bird
	3 birds in cage	minimum 550sq cm per bird
	4 birds in cage	minimum 430sq cm per bird
		minimum height of cage 35cm but at least 65% must be over 40cm high
		max. floor slope 14% on wire

Suggested maximum hen colony size 10,000. (Specific guidelines for different designations of chickens.)

Table Birds

Legal maximum stocking density	34kg bird-weight/sq metre 7lb per sq ft
Freedom Foods maximum	30kg bird-weight/sq metre

Transport Crates

Maximum bird weight per sq metre of crate	57kg
Minimum floor space per adult bird, according to weather	296–488sq cm

Minimum height, according to size of bird.

Birds less than 1.8kg bodyweight	220cm
Birds over 1.8kg bodyweight	255cm

Nests for Laying Birds

Minimum 1 nest per 5 birds.
Communal nests, minimum 1 sq metre nesting area per 80 hens.

Perch Length

Minimum 15cm per bird.

STOCKING DENSITIES (contd.)

Hours of Darkness

Minimum 6 hours, or hours of natural darkness in summer

Hours of Light

Minimum 8 hours
Recommended light intensity 20 lux (1 lux = 0.1 ft candle)

Access to Range

Minimum 8 hours, or hours of natural daylight in winter

Feeding Space

15cm per adult bird

Water Drinking Space

minimum 1 bell drinker per 80 birds

minimum length of trough available per adult bird 2.5cm

minimum 1 nipple per 10 hens

association between these problems and very rapid growth has been recognized by a number of marketing organizations that now require a controlled growth rate for all the chickens sold under their special quality designations.

- Foot lameness (Pododermatitis) and black hocks.
  These specific conditions indicate poor litter conditions, probably associated with overstocking and poor control of ventilation and temperature.
- Runting and stunting.
  This is a welfare problem if feeders and drinkers are raised too high for the smallest birds in an affected flock to reach. This management failure is often seen in practice.

Some guidelines and statistics on bird management are listed in the accompanying box.

Welfare Legislation

Welfare of Livestock. Miscellaneous Provisions Regulations 1968
Codes of Practice for the Welfare of Livestock 1987
Code of Practice for the Welfare of Poultry at Slaughter 1991
Welfare of Battery Hens Regulations 1993
Welfare of Livestock Regulations 1994
Welfare of Animals during Transport Regulations 1994
Freedom Foods RSPCA Standards 1995

8 The Multifactorial Nature of Disease —

One of the aims of this book is to show the fine balance that exists in nature between health and disease and to draw attention to the close relationship between the welfare of chickens and their health and resistance to disease, and therefore their ability to produce eggs or to grow into good table birds suitable for a quality market. Poultry are food animals and, apart from specialist pure-breed collections and backyard flocks, the chickens must constitute a part of an economically viable commercial flock. Their ability to produce eggs or grow into good table birds suitable for a quality market depends on their being in good health.

Often, several factors have to be involved before a disease can strike a poultry flock. If the number of these underlying contributory causes of any potential clinical disease outbreak is reduced by good management, the provision of a good environment for the poultry and a sensible veterinary policy for health control involving vaccinations and preventive medication, the chances of a flock being able to avoid clinical disease altogether and to be able to overcome any sudden new disease challenge correctly are greatly increased.

When a poultry flock meets a challenge from an infectious disease organism clearly defined factors determine whether the bird will be able to resist becoming clinically affected or whether it will succumb to serious disease. These factors include:

- The nature of the disease challenge.
- The weight of the disease challenge (the number of disease organisms challenging the chicken). (These are the qualitative and quantitative challenges.)
- The health of the chicken and the competence of its immune system.
- The standard of nutrition.
- The standard of management.
- The environment for the flock.
- The level of parasitic infection in the flock.
- The level of background environmental infection, for example, with E. Coli. clostridia, or staphylococci present in the house or in the water supply.
- Sub-clinical infection with other organisms already present in the birds, for example with mycoplasma, infectious bronchitis, turkey rhinotracheitis.
- The presence of any other stress factors that will predispose the flock to disease.

The environmental conditions for the flock influence the facility with which disease organisms present can multiply and cause serious clinical disease. High stocking density, poor hygiene and poor ventilation all increase the ability and speed with which introduced infections can spread through a flock. No flock, particularly those on extensive, multi-age and multi-hybrid poultry farms, can live in the complete absence of potential disease-producing organisms. These include mites, coccidia, parasites, bacteria and viruses. Good management of a flock must always

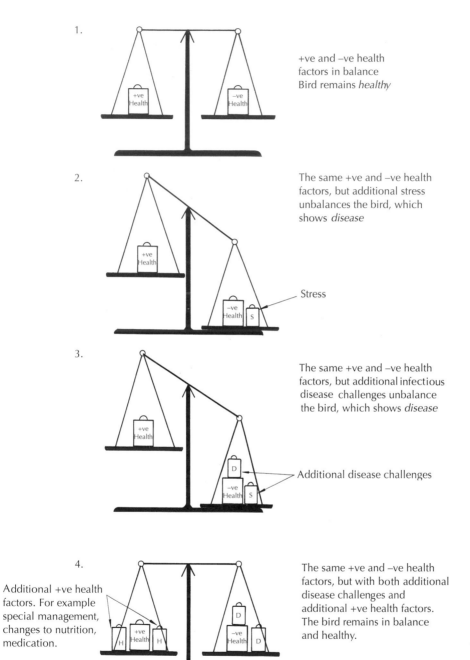

1. +ve and –ve health factors in balance Bird remains *healthy*

2. The same +ve and –ve health factors, but additional stress unbalances the bird, which shows *disease*

Stress

3. The same +ve and –ve health factors, but additional infectious disease challenges unbalance the bird, which shows *disease*

Additional disease challenges

4. The same +ve and –ve health factors, but with both additional disease challenges and additional +ve health factors. The bird remains in balance and healthy.

Additional +ve health factors. For example special management, changes to nutrition, medication.

Fig. 31
The balance between health and disease.

aim not for the complete absence of all infections but to maintain the balance between health and clinical disease in the chickens at all times.

Primary and Secondary Infections

While birds are suffering from a clinical disease they are more susceptible to other infections and these can prolong and complicate the original disease outbreak. This is what is meant by a primary and secondary infection. It must therefore be a principal of good management of any poultry flock to reduce the number of possible disease challenges and the weight of each challenge as much as possible. This should be part of normal management policy for the farm and will include:

- Stress-free management.
- Vaccination.
- Preventive medication.
- A disease break between crops.
- Unit security.
- A high standard of hygiene.

9 Nutrition and Nutritional Diseases

There is a wide variety of conditions affecting the health of poultry that are related to nutrition, ranging from sudden death caused by contamination of the food with fungal toxins, through the classical nutritional deficiencies that are described in all the text books to minor failures in bird growth rate or egg production. In fact nutrition should always be considered as being one of the possible factors contributing to a health problem except in the most obvious cases of infectious disease.

Farmers always find it very easy to 'blame the food' for a production or health problem of any kind in a flock. It is essential that, if they genuinely think the food may be involved in their problem, they contact the feed company and their vet immediately and also take a 2kg sample of the food that was being eaten at the time the symptoms first developed so that the problem can be fully investigated.

Except for broilers that are fed on highly specialized rations that provide for their very rapid growth and early slaughter as table birds all chickens should receive insoluble grit from an early age. This helps to develop the muscular power of the developing gizzard and enables the bird to grind up fibrous material that it could otherwise not digest.

DISEASES ASSOCIATED WITH NUTRITION IN CHICKS AND GROWING BIRDS

Problems in Baby Chicks and the Importance of the Parent Breeder Hen

Problems include failure of eggs to hatch, gross abnormalities in newly hatched chicks and poor variable or abnormal early development of the chicks. If a poultry farmer encounters any of these problems a full investigation should be made without delay. The maxim 'once a problem flock, always a problem flock' is usually true for a flock of chickens unless action can be taken quickly.

Before hatching, the developing chick is dependent on the food store in the egg and this in turn is dependent on the nutrition of the parent hen before the fertile egg was laid. The standard of commercial breeder rations varies widely, often for reasons of cost, and faults in milling and in the quality of the raw materials also occur occasionally. If the food is deficient in vital nutrients for the developing embryo the developing chicks may either not hatch at all, will be weak at hatching or will show clear signs of specific deficiencies during the first few days of life before they can eat enough of their chick starter ration to remedy any deficiencies. Abnormalities include thickening of the oesophagus and membranes in the mouth, abnormal down and feather development, curled toes, early nervous signs or weakness. These conditions are quite frequently seen in pure-breed collections where the breeder birds are kept in close confinement and feed on home designed rations. Some of the fed components often included in poultry rations are deficient in certain nutrients, for example maize and brassicas. On the other hand, when breeder hens are on traditional free range and can forage for a variety of food, deficiencies are much less likely. For hens not on range it is important that a correctly balanced vitamin and mineral supplement is added to their ration.

After the baby chick has hatched the quality of the food given to it is vitally important. All poultry farmers should start their chicks on a good-quality balanced starter crumb that contains all the nutritional factors required and whose digestibility is assured. Additionally, vitamin supplementation in the drinking water with a soluble high-quality product recommended by the vet is often beneficial for the first week of life. In chicks suspected of having deficiencies at the time they hatch, supplementation with the specifically required vitamins at high dose rate in the drinking water is, of course, essential.

Poor or Variable Early Growth of Chicks

This may be caused by disease, management or even the genetic make-up of pure breeds that have been close bred, but possible nutritional factors include:

- Dusty unpalatable starter crumbs that reduce the essential early food intake.
- The colour of the starter crumb.
  If there is no contrast between it and the floor under the chicks (corrugated paper, shavings, sawdust, and so on)

the chicks cannot distinguish between the food and the litter. This is a common reason for poor early food consumption. In addition to a change in the type of early crumb given, a change in the early bedding can be made or the lights can be relocated so that they shine more directly on the feed particles.
- The size of the crumb or starter pellets. This can be a problem in small breeds like bantams where the pellet may be too big for the bird to swallow. This is very often the case with game bird rations. It may occur in poultry if chicks have been severely beak trimmed. In any case food intake will be reduced.
- The nutritional content of the feed. It is obvious that this is an essential factor.

Poor Feathering, Aggression and Feather Eating

Late feathering is usually the result of chicks being kept at a high temperature for too long. Abnormal feathering, particularly when the developing feathers break at the shaft and stick out from the body (so called helicopter feathers), is usually the result of early virus infection, but nutritional deficiencies may also be involved. Shortage of vitamin B components in the ration and of sulphur-containing amino acids in the protein may be implicated. Feathers contain a lot of sulphur and poor-quality protein is often deficient in the expensive amino acids that contain sulphur. These amino acids are more concentrated in protein of animal origin and in suspected cases an analysis of the protein in the feed should be carried out with a view to adding the necessary synthetic acids, as is commonly done for intensively reared pigs. Poor feathering or the presence of loose or broken feathers is often associated with aggressive behaviour in the chicks. Nutritional deficiency will cause active feather eating and this will also precipitate an outbreak of aggression.

Nervous Signs in Young Chicks

Vitamin E deficiency causes a condition that used to be called crazy chick disease. In severe cases chicks cannot stand, have abnormal head movements, convulsions and spasms. Less severely affected birds show muscular weakness. It may be seen in chicks soon after hatching in which case the food of the parent breeder was probably deficient in the vitamin. When seen in birds over two weeks old the cause is a deficiency or non-availability of vitamin E in the starter food, probably because of rancidity. A virus condition, epidemic tremor, causes rather similar signs and the vet will be needed to establish the diagnosis. Both conditions are only seen in chicks less than four weeks old.

Clogging of the Beak and Mouth with Food and Distension of the Crop

This is quite often seen when the food is too creamy and low in fibre. The birds cannot swallow this and it accumulates in the back of the mouth. Other causes of clogging of the beak are described in Ch. 13.

Sudden Death of Chicks in Good Condition

A condition associated with nutrition can cause sudden death in well-grown broiler-type chicks between two and four weeks old. This is fatty liver kidney syndrome. The disease is related to a deficiency of biotin and the balance between carbohydrate and fat in the ration. The condition is readily diagnosed at post-mortem examination. Chicks are always well grown and the liver and kidneys are pale and often greasy. The carcass may be rather pinker than normal, in fact, the condition was originally called Pink Disease, before the cause was established. Treatment must include not only biotin but an adjustment to the ration and poultry farmers should seek advice on how to limit the condition in subsequent batches of birds that they rear.

Diarrhoea and Wet Litter

Nutritional factors causing this may include:

- excess salt in the feed;
- toxins and poisons;
- mouldiness of the feed;
- rancidity;
- the presence of too much added fat;
- too low fibre;
- feed of the wrong formulation being given to the chickens;
- poor quality ingredients, for example, excess tapioca.

There are many reasons for enteric disturbances in chickens and often several factors are involved.

Leg Weakness and Paralysis

Infections or specific toxins may be responsible but nutritional factors involving calcium, phosphorus and vitamin D3 must always be considered.

Rickets and Pseudorickets

The bones of the baby chick are elastic at hatching but in a healthy bird they should have calcified and become rigid before the bird is two weeks old. If there is a failure in calcification the bird becomes unable to sustain its increasing weight and goes off its legs – a post-mortem examination is necessary to establish the diagnosis. Mildly affected birds show bowing of the developing limb bones. All affected birds have flexible rubbery beaks that are unable to pick up food adequately when pecking. Causes include:

70

- Absolute deficiency of calcium in the feed.
- Gross excess of phosphorus in the ration.
- Deficiency of vitamin D3.
  This vitamin is not very stable and is destroyed by heat. Many cases of rickets seen in veterinary practice respond dramatically to additional vitamin D3 given in the drinking water.
- Early virus infection causing malabsorption.

Calcium carefully balanced with phosphorus should be given with additional vitamin D3 in the drinking water as a standard part of the treatment, but the underlying cause of the conditions must be established.

White Staining of the Vent and Death from Kidney Failure

Kidney diseases are described in Ch. 15.
One cause is a fault in nutrition. Rations for laying hens contain approximately 4 per cent of calcium to provide for mineralization of the eggshell but this amount is toxic for all chickens that are not laying eggs. These need a maximum of only 1 per cent calcium in the ration and if birds of any age are supplied in error with a layer bird ration they quickly suffer from kidney failure.

NUTRITIONAL PROBLEMS OF ADULT BIRDS

Paralysis, Brittle Bones and Poor Eggshell Quality in Hens

These are described in Chapters on reproductive diseases. Calcium and phosphorus levels, vitamin D3 and the provision of soluble calcium grit are all important nutritional factors in addition to the type of management under which the flock is kept. The magnesium content of feed can also affect eggshell quality.

Pallor and Sudden Death from Haemorrhage

This is seen in hens in high production and the cause may relate to nutrition. Hens of some breeds that are kept in cages or small coops have no chance to exercise. If they are fed high-energy low protein rations they can become excessively fat and this may cause fatty degeneration and haemorrhage in the liver (see Fig. 32). This either causes sudden death or sudden anaemia in the birds. An excess of rapeseed in the meal also causes a rather similar condition. Affected birds are either found suddenly dead or very pale and weak from massive internal haemorrhage.

Possible Nutritional Problems in Birds on Home-Produced and Organic Rations

Some marketing organizations for quality chicken specify that only vegetable protein may be given in the feed. In nature however chickens are omnivorous. They search out and eat animal protein in the form of earthworms, beetles and other invertebrates and also accidentally eat all the small animal organisms, for example aphids, that live on the plants that are part of their normal ration. The number of these creatures becomes greatly depleted in paddocks that are rotationally grazed by hens on tightly managed free-range systems, particularly when the paddocks are ploughed up and resown with simple rye grass mixtures. Birds on range of this kind therefore do not have the opportunity of consuming large amounts of animal protein. Animal protein contains a different mix of amino acids from vegetable protein and deficiencies sometimes

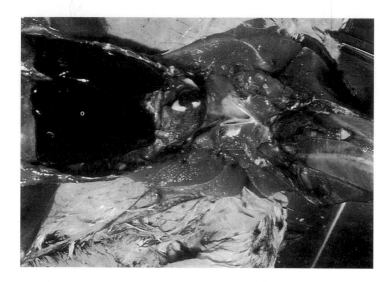

Fig. 32 Internal haemorrhage. The abdomen is full of clotted blood.

show in birds on strictly vegetable protein diets. The clinical signs include poor feathering, dry dull feathers, compulsive feather eating by the birds and cannibalism as well as egg production failures. The amount of 'protein' in a ration is not the most vital consideration in choosing a ration for chickens. The digestibility of protein from different raw material varies widely according both to the type and quality, and the amounts of the different essential amino acids in it also varies widely. It is these factors, among others, that determine the real value of a food.

SOME POSSIBLE FAULTS IN THE QUALITY OF COMMERCIAL FEEDS

- A computer error at the mill has led to an alteration in the ration specification.
- Incompatibility of ration ingredients in a computerized Least-Cost ration formulation.
- Contamination of the feed with a different ration at the mill.
  For example a pullet ration is contaminated with a layer ration that was the previous one milled.

- The wrong ration delivered to the farm.
- Dustiness of the feed or variation in crumb size.
  This affects palatability and allows for separation of ingredients and selection by the birds. If whole grain is present this may be picked out by some of the birds and the rest of the feed rejected.
- Pellet size and colour.
  This can affect palatability.
- The quality of raw materials.
  Affects digestibility and production.
- Poor storage after milling.
  May cause rancidity, mould growth and toxicity, degradation of vitamins and poor palatability.
- Overheating during milling.
  Causes inactivation of vitamins, particularly vitamin D3. Also an effect on colour, palatability and nutrient value of the feed.

POISONS AND TOXINS

The symptoms that birds show in outbreaks of poisoning are not always distinctive and are often difficult to differentiate from infectious disease. They may vary from sudden death or paralysis to incoordination or other nervous signs, diarrhoea, thirst or dehydration, or more chronic illthrift and drops in production.

Chickens can be poisoned in the following ways:

- By pecking poisonous plants or other materials on the farm.
- By eating a contaminated or incorrect ration.
- By drinking contaminated water.
- By absorption through the skin.
- In the air that they breathe.

It is good practice for a farmer to keep an up-to-date list of the substances that are commonly present on his farm that are known to be poisonous. These can be considered first if a suspected poisoning incident ever occurs. It is most important to involve the vet without delay if poisoning is ever implicated in a disease problem, particularly if the feed is involved. He can then give the necessary expert evidence if a claim for damages has to be made or a court case brought later on. Accurate laboratory diagnosis often has to depend on chemical analysis which is very expensive. If the poultry farmer and his vet work together in the investigation of a problem they should be able to narrow down the number of possible causes and therefore the cost of the analyses that have to be made.

Poisonous Substances That May be Present on a Farm

- *Poisonous Plants.*
Many plants can cause poisoning but the following are amongst the most likely to be present:

Rhubarb and daffodils
Cause diarrhoea.

Laburnum, hemlock and water hemlock
Cause incoordination and convulsions.

Yew
Can cause collapse and death although chickens will actually rarely eat it.

Green potatoes
These are very poisonous and cause incoordination, paralysis and diarrhoea.

- *Disinfectants based on phenol, and wood that has been painted with creosote.*
These cause inappetence and thirst, and taints in poultry carcasses and eggs and they may also be absorbed through the skin.

- *Rat Baits*
The potentiated warfarin baits are very poisonous and can cause death with diarrhoea and haemorrhage. Chickens are very resistant to simple warfarin baits.

- *Agricultural Chemicals.*

Insecticides and herbicides
Organophosphorus and organochlorine products. These cause nervous signs and diarrhoea or non-specific illness.

Alphachloralos for pigeon control.
This is very poisonous for chickens and causes coma and death.

Metaldehyde for slug control.
Some chickens will actively seek out slug pellets, which will cause incoordination and narcosis.

Litter
Hardwood shavings can contain dactylaria or fungicides which may cause incoordination.

- *Mouldy Food and Bedding*
These may contain fungal toxins. Signs of poisoning are usually chronic. Birds become unthrifty and egg production is reduced. There may be diarrhoea.

- *Botulinus toxin.*

Botulism is caused by a very potent toxin that causes loss of muscular power, paralysis and death in chickens of all ages. The toxin is produced by bacteria that can be present in rotting carcasses and muddy effluents. When these, or the maggots or small invertebrate animals that feed on them, are eaten by the bird poisoning follows. Occasionally the toxin can be present in commercial meat and bone or blood meal. The course of the disease is very rapid and there is no treatment. The birds' muscles become quite flaccid and they are unable even to raise their heads. Some die from respiratory failure. Diagnosis is not easy to confirm and advice should be sought from the vet immediately a problem is recognized.

- *Arsenic, copper, phosphorus, strychnine, zinc phosphide and mercury.*

These traditional poisons are now seldom used but stocks may still be present on a farm. Symptoms in poisoned birds vary from convulsions and death to diarrhoea and liver and kidney failure and diagnosis by chemical analysis is usually necessary.

- *Accidental overdose with medicines, or incompatibilities between medicines being given simultaneously.*

Substances in Commercial Poultry Feeds That May Cause Poisoning

The demarcation line between a fault in the 'quality' of food delivered and presence of 'poison' is a fine one, because an excessive amount of most of the inclusions in commercial feeds, for instance, minerals, trace elements, vitamins or other additives, is toxic. In any cases where poisoning is suspected a 2kg sample of the food being given at the time symptoms were first shown should be taken. This should be sealed in a plastic bag to exclude as much air as possible and fully identified with the type of ration, delivery date and any other relevant information.

Substances to consider are:

- Excess salt.
- Causes thirst and diarrhoea, and in serious cases paralysis and death.
- Excess magnesium.
  This can cause poor eggshell quality and brittle bones in hens.
- Excess calcium in rations given to chickens that are not laying eggs.
  Normal layer rations that contain 4 per cent calcium needed for eggshell production may cause death from kidney failure if fed accidentally to other birds.
- Excess rapeseed oil.
  This will cause taint in eggs and death in hens from liver degeneration and haemorrhage.
- Tallow and other toxic fats.
  These can cause death and post-mortem examination will show oedema of the carcass.
- Excess Ionophore Coccidiostats.
  These can cause panting, muscular weakness, paralysis and death, particularly in rapidly growing table chickens that have an opportunity to overeat.
- Fungal toxins.
  These cause illthrift, diarrhoea and poor egg production and predispose affected birds to other diseases.

Poisoning of Chickens through Absorption through the Skin

- Insecticides, particularly organophosphorous chemicals.
  These are very poisonous to chickens which may show nervous symptoms, paralysis and death if the compounds are sprayed directly onto them.
- Phenolic disinfectants and creosote.
  These are absorbed through the skin and severe poisoning can result from

this route. Poisoning from this cause is quite commonly seen on traditional farms where disinfection and painting has been carried out with these products. In mild cases the meat and eggs are tainted by the disinfectant.

Poisons in Contaminated Water

In Britain the most likely contaminants are disinfectants, sheep-dips and other insecticides, and lead. Otherwise poisoning is rare except after industrial accidents. In some countries water supplies contain high concentrations of minerals and may be toxic in their own right.

Poisoning from the Air (Environmental Poisoning)

Poultry farmers must remember that chickens are often poisoned if the air in the poultry house is polluted either because the ventilation is poor or because gas equipment is burning incorrectly. The levels of oxygen, carbon monoxide, carbon dioxide and ammonia in a poultry house can be regularly checked quite easily and inexpensively using a Draeger kit.

- Ammonia
  Ammonia fumes produced from the breakdown of droppings build up during the time a poultry house is shut up or when the fans are turned off at night in order to keep the temperature up. This can occur in both littered houses and laying houses with droppings pits under the floor slats. Ammonia can also build up in areas of 'dead air' between fans, or from litter that has become damp and is not working properly.
  If poisoning is suspected a round-the-clock monitoring of the quality of the air at bird level (the air that the chickens are actually breathing) is necessary before the possibility of ammonia build-

up in a poultry house can be eliminated. Air must always be sampled at bird level because poisonous gases tend to layer in a house according to their density. Excess ammonia in the air can usually be detected by the poultryman and an exact measurement can be made using the Draeger kit. The maximum amount of ammonia permitted in the air under Health and Safety at Work Legislation is 5ppm. The symptoms of ammonia poisoning are described in detail in the chapter on the eye.

- Carbon monoxide
  This is always extremely poisonous, both to chickens and to the poultry attendants, causing failure in oxygen exchange and rapid coma and death. Carcasses of dead birds are a noticeably brighter red colour than normal. The cause is faulty burning of gas appliances and this may be the result of either restricted ventilation or a fault in the machine. It is of the utmost importance, for the health and safety of both staff and poultry, that all gas appliances are regularly checked to ensure that they are burning correctly, and also that gas is never used in a building with restricted ventilation.

- Carbon dioxide
  This builds up in poultry houses with high stocking rates for the chickens and/or large numbers of gas burners in the house if ventilation is inadequate. High levels cause respiratory distress and predispose birds to disease.

- Formalin
  This has been used to disinfect nesting boxes and the fumes occasionally cause respiratory distress and conjunctivitis. If used in a hatchery it also poison the developing chicks.

- Dust
  Excessive amounts of dust in the air predispose birds to respiratory and other diseases. The maximum amount

of dust permitted in the air in a building under the Health and Safety at Work Legislation is 10mg per cubic metre of air.

Control

The vet will recommend specific treatment for an individual outbreak. Immediate emergency measures should ensure that the birds have plenty of fresh water to drink, preferably medicated with an electrolyte solution, and all food should be removed immediately. If gas poisoning is suspected burners and ventilation should be checked.

After a poisoning incident special treatment may have to be given to aid recovery and this may include a special diet or vitamin supplementation. The subsequent progress of an affected flock should be carefully recorded in case there is a consequential loss and the progress of the flock must be monitored by the farmer's veterinary surgeon, whose certification will always be required if any claim for damages is brought.

Gas Poisoning Levels

Gas	Permitted by Legislation	Level at which poisoning is likely
Ammonia	5ppm	over 30 is always potentially poisonous
Carbon Monoxide	50ppm	No additional tolerance
Carbon Dioxide	500ppm	No additional tolerance

10 The Immune System ━━━━━━━

IMMUNITY AND RESISTANCE TO INFECTION

All poultry keepers should have a general understanding of what immunity to disease means, and how it develops in the chickens on their farms. Resistance to infection is vital for the survival of the chickens whenever they meet a disease challenge during their lives and the success or failure of a vaccination programme that is given to a flock also depends on an appreciation of what the vaccines are trying to achieve, and how vaccines differ from 'medicines'.

The immune system of the chicken consists of concentrations of lymphoid cells of different types with complex interacting functions that help to protect the bird from infections. The cells are divided into two classes (B or T cells) that become modified to carry out specific functions. Some actually produce antibodies that are complex chemicals that can act on and neutralize specific disease-producing organisms. The function of other cells is to recognize infections and stimulate the production of antibody. Others are memory cells that store information about infections that the bird meets for future use in producing immunity. Still others act like soldiers and actively hunt out and destroy the living organisms that cause disease. As always in nature, the complexity of a living animal is incredible and

makes even the most advanced computer seem relatively simple.

The cells of the immune system are found in a number of separate locations in the chicken. They can be studied by a pathologist during a careful post-mortem examination and their appearance can often give an indication of the efficiency of the immune system in the particular bird. It is not necessary for a poultry owner to go into more detail but for readers interested an outline of the anatomy of the immune system is given in the appendix to this chapter.

A baby chick has a partly functional immune system by the time it hatches. However, it is extremely susceptible to a number of serious diseases as soon as it has hatched and these diseases can kill it before its immune system has been able to react. Nature has guarded against this to some extent because the baby chick can derive a temporary immunity to some, but not all, of these diseases from its egg yolk in the same way that a new-born calf can derive immunity from its mother's milk. This can only happen against diseases that the parent hen has actually experienced. If her immune system is fully functional it produces antibodies against these diseases and these diffuse in the yolk of each egg that she produces in her ovary. The antibodies are then instantly available for the chick when it hatches but they degenerate after two or three weeks. The effectiveness of this temporary immunity varies

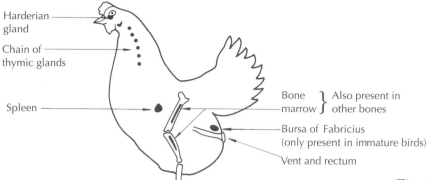

Harderian gland

Chain of thymic glands

Spleen

Bone marrow } Also present in other bones

Bursa of Fabricius (only present in immature birds)

Vent and rectum

Fig. 33   Location of the main centres of immune tissue.

widely in individual eggs because of a number of factors.

By making use of both the transfer of this temporary immunity from the hen and the chick's own immune system it has been possible, in recent years, to develop vaccines against many of the diseases that affect baby chicks. This now makes it possible to rear chicks successfully in very large numbers on poultry farms even when some serious infections are present.

THE ANATOMY OF THE IMMUNE SYSTEM IN THE CHICKEN

The Bursa of Fabricius is a small almost spherical creamy/grey-coloured organ situated dorsal to the rectum at the vent. It has a folded glandular lining and consists of B-lymphocytes. It is the most important location of immune tissue in the young chicken but shrinks and becomes dysfunctional as the bird matures. It is specifically attacked and destroyed by Gumboro disease virus.

There is also a concentration of immune tissue in the neck. This is the bird's thymus and appears as a loosely connected string of small pinkish grey nodules on either side of the neck alongside the windpipe and oesophagus.

The spleen, a small rounded organ purplish in colour situated between the liver and the gizzard also contains large numbers of lymphoid cells and the bone marrow is also important.

A small gland behind the eye, the Harderian gland, is also an important

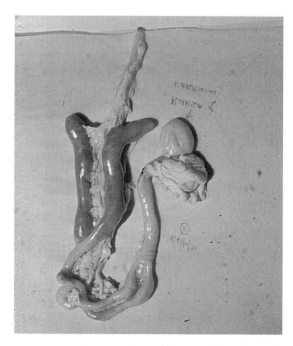

Fig. 34   The Bursa of Fabricius

immune organ and produces antibody to infections that reach the eye. This function is utilized when certain live vaccines are given to chickens by eye drop (Ch. 25).

There are other smaller concentrations of immune tissue throughout the chicken's body and all these areas contribute to the ability of the bird to resist infection or other damage.

DISEASES AFFECTING THE IMMUNE SYSTEM

Some disease organisms in chickens directly attack and destroy cells in the immune system. The most important of these are Gumboro disease and chicken anaemia virus. Diseases of this kind not only affect the chicken directly and cause illness and mortality but, by destroying part of their immune system, they leave surviving birds with a reduced ability to overcome other diseases and often unable to develop a satisfactory immunity after the vaccination. In this way they have similarities with the AIDS virus that affects human beings. In addition to these specific infections a large number of other diseases also reduce the efficiency of the immune system more indirectly. Examples are Mareks disease, avian rhinotracheitis (ART), aspergillosis (brooder pneumonia) and poisoning from fungal toxins (aflatoxins).

Chickens that have survived the acute stage of any of these diseases often remain unthrifty. If sacrificed for a port-mortem examination the pathologist will find a significant reduction in the amount of immune tissue present in them.

GUMBORO DISEASE

It is important for all poultry farmers who rear chickens of any type to be able to recognize and understand this disease that affects the subsequent development and performance of most affected flocks. It can also cause sudden drops in egg production in laying birds that are still susceptible.

Gumboro disease is caused by a virus and there are different strains that cause disease of different levels of severity. The virus is very resistant and will remain alive for over a year in the dusty environment of a poultry unit. It also infects litter beetles, fomites and other creatures. These act as intermediate hosts and can keep the organism alive for long periods of time. On an infected farm it is essential to reduce the amount of infection before another flock is reared in the same building and a very rigorous sanitization programme between each flock of chickens is essential. The hygiene programme must include all the areas *outside* the poultry houses as well as the houses themselves because the virus will have contaminated these areas in the dusty air extracted from the poultry house during the life of the chickens and in the litter removed from the house after they have gone. Maintenance of the poultry houses between crops is also important in order to reduce the number of places where insects can breed. This must be combined with the use of effective insecticidal sprays. On multi-age farms the elimination of the infection will have to be done progressively over a year or so.

On farms where there is only one age of bird being reared at any one time the disease usually comes on quite suddenly when the chickens are between 25 and 35 days of age. The birds become dull and there is mortality which may reach 20 per cent. The disease rapidly affects the kidneys and the vents of some birds often become stained with white evil-smelling urate material. Deaths are often quite sudden and dead birds are found on their sides. An epidemic usually lasts for about a week but after this the surviving birds often remain unthrifty and are also very susceptible to a number of other infections.

On multi-age farms or farms where the standard of hygiene is poor chicks may become infected much earlier. Pullets being reared for egg production are particularly susceptible. Chicks that become infected before they are three weeks old do not show any typical symptoms but their immune system is even more severely damaged than when older birds are affected. The birds become unthrifty and often die later from other diseases.

On farms where young chicks have some degree of immunity from the parent breeders the disease may show only as poor growth and variable condition in the birds when they are between five and twelve weeks old. Affected birds often have persistent diarrhoea.

Birds that have had Gumboro disease are often unable to develop an immunity after the vaccinations that are part of their normal rearing programme, for example to infectious bronchitis and Newcastle disease. This is because the virus has destroyed part of their immune system.

A post-mortem examination must always be carried out by the vet to confirm a diagnosis of Gumboro disease. Typically, acutely affected birds show changes in the Bursa of Fabricius, kidney damage and dehydration, often with the accumulation of white urate material in the ureters and tissues.

Control

On all poultry farms the control of Gumboro disease must be by a combination of good hygiene and vaccination; vaccination on its own is not enough. Vaccine must be given before the chicks become infected and the type of vaccine used must depend on the virulence of the strain of Gumboro disease virus present and the level of infection on the farm. The temporary immunity passed on by the parent breeders if they have been vaccinated is also an important tool in the difficult control of this disease.

Treatment

As with all virus diseases the virus itself cannot be killed with drugs but the severity of an outbreak can often be reduced significantly by treatment to increase the water consumption of the birds and by the use of electrolytes and possibly a change of food.

CHICKEN ANAEMIA VIRUS

This virus also causes serious disease in young chickens of any type, usually when the birds are between two and six weeks old.

The poultryman will first notice that the flock is becoming uneven and that some birds are obviously sick. Mortality will rise and often deaths from general E. coli or other infections, including coccidiosis, occur. Veterinary diagnosis on n post-mortem shows anaemia and the bone marrow appears a characteristic creamy pink instead of its normal strong redcurrant jelly colour. Affected birds often also show secondary bacterial infection and there are other typical lesions that are described in avian pathology textbooks.

The way in which chicks become infected with this virus is complex but usually involves transmission from the parent flocks in a few chicks and later spreads from chick to chick. Chicks should receive an effective immunity via the egg and by the time they are six weeks old healthy chicks are no longer susceptible to the disease. However, if their immune system has been damaged by infection with some other disease, particularly Gumboro disease or Mareks disease, they remain susceptible to the disease for much longer and chicken anaemia virus has recently become one of the most troublesome problems for poultry farmers.

Control of the disease for all types of chicken is by blood testing and vaccination of breeder flocks. This is very successful if it is carried out correctly under the supervision of the vet.

Treatment

As with all virus infections there is no effective specific treatment but vitamin supplementation, a ration with an increased nutrient value and the control of secondary infections all help to improve the growth of an affected flock.

11 The Musculo-skeletal System —

SKELETON, MUSCLES AND JOINTS

The primary function of the bony skeleton is to provide a rigid frame for the growing bird that enables it to develop to its full potential. It also provides the attachments for the muscles, tendons and ligaments that enable the bird to move and carry out normal activity.

An additional function of the bones in the laying hen is to make possible the rapid calcium exchange in the bird's body that is necessary to lay down the shell each time the bird produces an egg. See Ch. 22.

Chickens reared for meat production have a genetic potential for very rapid growth, particularly of breast muscle. A day-old chick that weighs 40gm can weigh over 2kg by the time it is six weeks old. At some stages of its development a broiler chicken can convert more than half the energy value of the food it eats into an increase in body weight. This is what is meant by a Food Conversion Rate of Two (FCR2).

For a poultry farmer to grow this type of chicken successfully the management of the flock must be of a very high standard. If it is not, the strength of the bird's skeleton may not keep up with its increasing weight and the legs of the rapidly growing bird will not be able to fully support it. The bird will become lame, unable to walk, and increasingly suscep-tible to other diseases. The incidence of this type of lameness is greatly influenced by the background levels of disease in the flock, for example with E. coli, salmonella, staphylococcus, mycoplasma and certain viruses.

- The chicks should be healthy at day old and have no hereditary weaknesses.
- They should be active right through their growing period; exercise is essential for optimum development of bones, joints and muscles in all types of chickens.
- The environment should be comfortable for the birds and the flock well super-vised.
- They should be fed on a correctly bal-anced feed programme.
- The birds should be reared in the absence of infections, all of which are setbacks to optimum growth.

Genetic Faults

Some locomotor diseases are breed-related and occur in particular bloodlines of birds. The primary breeding companies work progressively to reduce these conditions.

They include:

- Tibial dyschondroplasia (TD).
This is a failure in the development of the cartilage in the leg bones, particularly the tibia, in rapidly growing broiler type chickens. It only causes lameness in severely affected birds but affects the later growth of birds kept on as roasters.

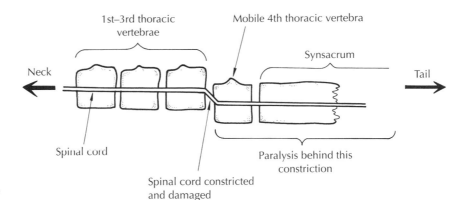

Fig. 35 Kinky back.

- Deformed toes.

Some chicks have deformed toes when they hatch. This can be breed-related. Other deformities are caused by faults in nutrition. However, often the condition is management-related and this can develop in any type of chicken. If the birds are kept under conditions where they cannot use their toes to grip and perch, the feet do not develop normally and the toes become progressively deformed as the birds get older. This condition is commonly seen in older roaster chickens and in laying hens that have been reared intensively.

- Kinky back.

This is a paralytic condition seen in broiler chickens when they are about a month old. Birds are found lying on their sides

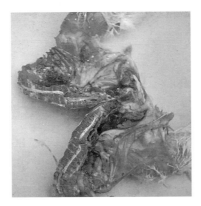

*Fig. 36
Kinky back.*

and are quite unable to stand. Only the legs and posterior part of the bird are affected, the bird appears bright and the wings, head and neck are normal. The cause is a dislocation of the last free thoracic vertebra in the back. This pinches the spinal cord and causes paralysis behind the injury.

TYPES OF LOCOMOTOR DISEASE

The poultry farmer should recognize particular symptoms in the birds and then work back to the possible causes.

Reluctance to Walk

- Disease of the hip.

This is the most common cause. Degeneration and infection of the hip joint and the top part of the femur is very common in meat chickens of all ages and also occurs occasionally in other breeds. It is one of the major disease problems in the poultry industry.

In all cases hip disease shows as a reluctance to walk. Some young affected chicks show dislocation of the hip. A large percentage of birds may be affected in a flock and the condition causes a serious welfare problem in the birds. The condition is being investigated in depth by

83

the poultry industry and agricultural research organizations under the guidance of the Farm Animal Welfare Council.

In many cases it is a developmental

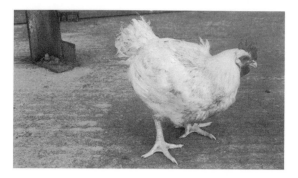

Fig. 37   Hip lameness (1). Bird standing leaning forward and unable to walk.

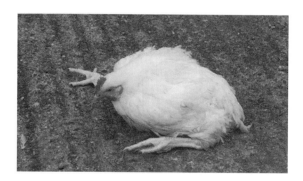

Fig. 38   Hip lameness (2). Advanced case, bird unable to stand without assistance.

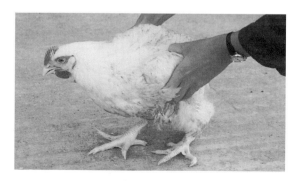

Fig. 39   Hip lameness (3). The bird in (2), standing with assistance.

failure and general infection is not present. In some, however, there is bacterial infection of the region, often with involvement of the bone marrow (osteomyelitis). Many meat chickens that die from other causes are found at post-mortem to have diseased hips. E. coli, salmonella and staphylococci are commonly involved and treatment with suitable antibiotics limits spread to some extent. If salmonella is found this presents a potential public health problem and, in Britain, must be notified by the diagnostic laboratory to government under the Zoonosis Order.

In many seriously affected flocks the cause is complex and multifactorial and not always fully understood. Both for welfare and economic reasons this type of lameness is very serious and a high incidence in any flock should always be fully investigated. Clearly, if cases are not discovered on the farm the quality of the carcass will be unacceptable. It must be stated, however, that it is not possible for a poultry meat inspector to spot all affected birds at the factory and broiler and roaster chickens with diseased hips commonly find their way onto the market. This is clearly unacceptable.

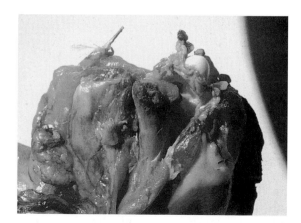

Fig. 40   Diseased hip in a broiler. (Femoral head necrosis.) This is the condition shown in photographs 37–9.

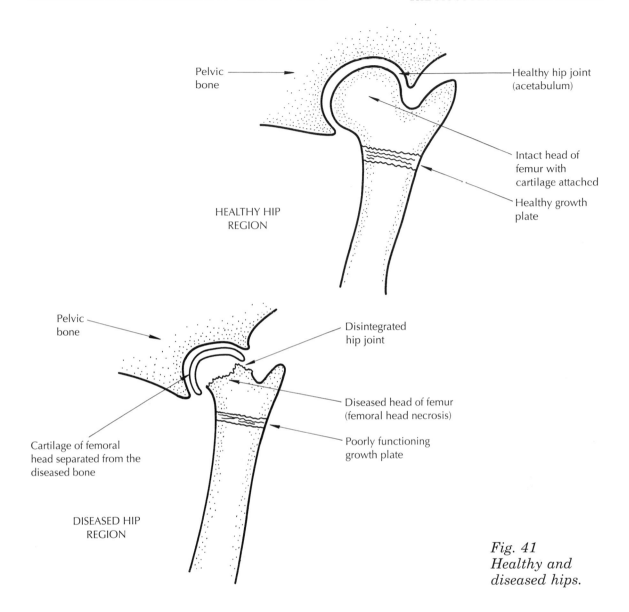

Pelvic bone

Healthy hip joint (acetabulum)

Intact head of femur with cartilage attached

Healthy growth plate

HEALTHY HIP REGION

Pelvic bone

Disintegrated hip joint

Diseased head of femur (femoral head necrosis)

Poorly functioning growth plate

Cartilage of femoral head separated from the diseased bone

DISEASED HIP REGION

Fig. 41
Healthy and
diseased hips.

● Rickets

Young chickens with any form of rickets are also reluctant to walk. The term rickets is loosely used to describe any failure in the proper calcification of the bones in developing chicks between the ages of about ten days and six weeks. The bones remain elastic and will bend without snapping. The beak is also pliable which makes the chick unable to pick up food effectively. Although the chicks remain looking bright the condition rapidly develops in some birds so that they cannot stand and the poultryman may think the birds are paralysed. If it is thought that faulty nutrition may be the cause of the problem a food sample should be taken and retained for later analysis if required. In addition to nutritional causes, failure of the skeleton to calcify is often seen in any breed of chick as a result of early infection with one of the group of viruses that causes infectious runting and stunting. These viruses reduce the absorption of nutrients during digestion and therefore cause nutritional deficiencies even when birds are on very good rations. These conditions are very serious in the poultry industry.

● Sore and Ulcerated Feet

These conditions are very common in broilers and roasters (see pp. 87–8). If the feet are severely ulcerated and if there is bacterial infection the birds become very reluctant to walk at all, but the condition shows up first as lameness and should be spotted at that stage by the poultryman.

It is usually a sign that the birds are being reared under unhygienic conditions, that the litter is poorly managed or that droppings are sticky and contaminating the birds' feet. When an affected bird is picked up the foot is usually caked in droppings. When these are pulled off the foot pad underneath is raw and ulcerated and often the whole foot is swollen and infected. Affected birds are lame and reluctant to move. In a badly affected flock infection spreads from the feet and deaths occur from general bacterial infection, usually either with E. coli or staphylococcus. Treatment with antibiotic, coupled with the necessary improvements to the environment, is successful, but care must be taken to comply with the withdrawal periods required for the antibiotic used before the birds can be slaughtered. Pullets reared under poor conditions can also suffer from this condition.

Paralysis

Paralysis is the end result of a number of quite separate conditions, but it is the one frequently seen by the poultryman. An accurate diagnosis will usually depend on post-mortem examinations and a careful assessment of the condition of the flock as a whole with the vet. An indication of some of the most common causes is given in the following list.

● Mareks disease in several of its forms can cause paralysis.
● Paralysis from brittle bone disease in laying hens is described in the chapter on conditions of the reproductive system.
● Chicks severely affected with any of the forms of rickets cannot stand and appear paralysed.
● Chicks with vitamin E deficiency may show general muscular weakness and be unable to stand but usually show nervous signs.
● Kinky back is described under genetic defects.
● Other paralytic conditions are described in the chapter on nervous diseases.

Swollen or Stiff Joints (Arthritis)

Affected joints are stiff causing obvious lameness and often pain. The affected areas are frequently hot and swollen. These typical signs of lameness can occur in chickens of all types and ages. The poultryman will readily spot them either in individual birds or as a flock problem in which case the vet should be contacted to discuss the cause and treatment. Individual birds should be separated from other birds in the flock and either culled or treated.

Causes include:

● Staphylococcal infection.
The hock joints are most commonly affected, also the feet when the condition is called bumblefoot. Infection often generalizes causing mortality in the flock. This infection often indicates a dirty environment for the chickens, often with rough surfaces in the poultry house that cause abrasions through which the bacteria can penetrate. Sharp

spicules of wood on perches, or worn and broken wire netting are common sites of entry for the bacteria.

- E. coli.
  This ubiquitous bacterium is associated with diseases of almost all kinds and commonly causes septic joints.
- Mycoplasma.
  Lameness caused by mycoplasma is now uncommon but is occasionally seen, particularly in pullet flocks between eight and eighteen weeks of age. The cause is usually *Mycoplasma synoviae*.

The poultryman will notice that a flock quite suddenly shows a number of lame birds and that the flock as a whole appears unwell. The birds may also be showing respiratory signs. Individual birds have soft swellings of the hocks and the feet and wing joints are also affected in some birds. This disease is very infectious and severely affects the subsequent development and performance of the flock so if it is suspected the vet must be contacted without delay. Treatment controls the symptoms in most birds but does not completely prevent the subsequent poor egg production in potential laying flocks. Furthermore, mycoplasmal infections always leave carrier birds in a flock even after treatment, so relapses are frequent. This is disastrous in a breeding flock because this is one of the group of diseases that passes from one generation to the next through the egg.

There are other types of arthritis but they are not so common. Heavy roasters may sometimes become acutely lame with a large swelling of a hock joint. The swelling quickly becomes dark red and later green and black. It is caused by haemorrhage under the skin from rupture of the main tendon to the foot (gastrocnemius). The cause is a virus (reovirus), against which vaccination is effective.

Fractures and Dislocations

- Fractures.
  Fractures in growing chickens are uncommon and only occur in individual birds as a result of accident. However, they are common in laying hens and if the incidence in a flock is high it is either because there is a failure in the calcium metabolism of the flock, or that the chicken house is badly designed and allows the birds to injure themselves. A thorough inspection of the house should be made to establish where the injuries are occurring. Pullets that have been reared under very intensive conditions with little exercise are much more liable to injury than birds that are more rugged by the time they are at point of lay. In all affected flocks extra attention to the provision of calcium, phosphorus, vitamin D3 and grit must be given. Any bird with a fracture must be removed from the flock and individually treated or culled.

- Dislocations.
  Except for those in individual birds that are the result of injury, dislocations are only found in growing birds. They are very common in broiler flocks, particularly in birds about three weeks old. One or both hocks will be seen to be sticking out at an angle from the upper part of the leg. The bird is unable to walk and must be culled on welfare grounds immediately. There is no effective treatment.

The cause may be a developmental failure with twisting of the developing bones that allows the tendons to slip sideways, but it is often an indication of the presence of an underlying disease problem in the flock. This may be runting and stunting, chicken anaemia virus, gumboro disease, salmonella or E. coli infection. As with other multifactorial conditions a thorough investigation must be made to search for the primary cause of the problem.

In baby chicks dislocation of the hip occurs in birds with spraddle legs, in some with hip lameness, and in some early cases of rickets.

Other Conditions

● Deformed toes.
The causes have been described under genetic defects.

● Burnt hocks.
This condition is usually found with pododermatitis and the cause is the same. A number of birds, usually in a broiler flock, have blackened or ulcerated areas just below the back of their hock joints where the leg is in contact with the litter when the bird lies down. Infection often spreads into the hock joint and may generalize, as in pododermatitis. Affected birds then become lame.

Both these conditions are diseases of bad management. If the official veterinary surgeon at a slaughterhouse finds cases he will notify the flock owner and should also contact the nominated veterinary surgeon for the poultry farm to check on the welfare of birds on the farm and make necessary recommendations.

● Bumblefoot.
Swelling and septicaemia of a foot without ulceration in individual birds is usually caused by staphylococcal infection.

Conditions affecting the musculoskeletal system have been considered in detail because of their importance to all poultry farmers, whether they are looking after very large units or just a few birds. Avoiding them is important for the welfare of flocks and welfare guidelines on poultry management give clear advice to all farmers on how to prevent the conditions that are management-related.

12 The Respiratory System ——————

The main function of the respiratory system is that of gaseous exchange; to absorb oxygen and excrete carbon dioxide. Its other function, that of temperature control, is less well known. A bird has no sweat glands and most of the body is insulated from rapid heat loss by the feathers. For rapid cooling it has to depend on the limited areas of skin that are bare and rich in blood vessels, the wattles and combs (and these are not well developed in some birds), and on the evaporation of water during breathing.

The structure of the respiratory system in birds differs in important ways from that of mammals and there are also wide variations between different species that relate to their evolution and lifestyle.

In the chicken the paired nostrils are located on the dorsal surface of the beak and lead to the complex nasal chambers that are folded and convoluted. Their highly vascular mucous lining assists both in warming the inhaled air and in removing dust particles which may contain infectious organisms from it. There is a pouch, the infra orbital sinus, that leads from the posterior end of the chamber and is located under the eye. This sinus is frequently involved in respiratory disease.

The nasal passages open into the posterior part of the mouth. If the bird breathes in with its beak open two airstreams converge, as they do in mammals, before the air passes through the cartilaginous larynx into the windpipe (trachea). The principal function of the larynx is to prevent food and water passing through it into the lungs; it does not actually produce the voice of the bird as is often thought.

The windpipe is a strong wide diameter tube strengthened with cartilaginous rings that leads down the neck to the entrance of the chest where it divides into two bronchi. At this point is another complex structure, the syrinx. This is the true voice organ of the chicken and consists of membranes reinforced with cartilage which can vibrate and produce sound like a musical instrument. The structure of the syrinx is specific to each species of bird, being modified in order to produce sounds as varied as that of the nightingale or the farmyard duck. Its structure is important to understand when considering respiratory disease because the windpipe reduces in diameter at the syrinx and this makes it the most probable place for blockage to occur. Both the trachea and bronchi are lined with a mixture of cells that secrete mucus (called goblet cells) and others that have numerous very fine short threads (cilia) that project into the lining of the respiratory pathway. The mucus traps dust particles and micro-organisms like bacteria, and the cilia beat continuously in rhythm setting up a current that projects the mucus and trapped detritus back up the windpipe to the mouth where it is either swallowed or coughed out. The successful functioning of this mechanism is vital to the bird and if it is upset by environ-

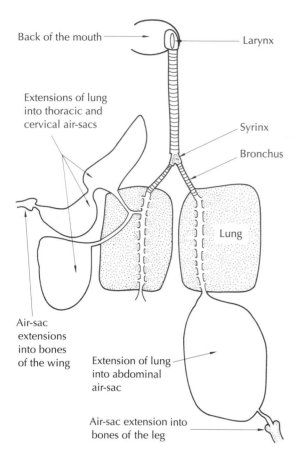

Back of the mouth — Larynx

Extensions of lung into thoracic and cervical air-sacs

Syrinx

Bronchus

Lung

Air-sac extensions into bones of the wing

Extension of lung into abdominal air-sac

Air-sac extension into bones of the leg

Fig. 42   The respiratory system.

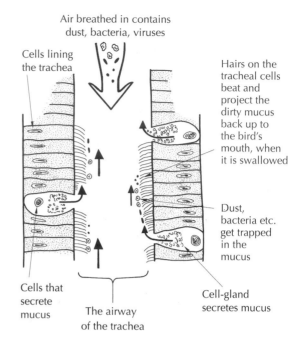

Air breathed in contains dust, bacteria, viruses

Cells lining the trachea

Hairs on the tracheal cells beat and project the dirty mucus back up to the bird's mouth, when it is swallowed

Dust, bacteria etc. get trapped in the mucus

Cells that secrete mucus

The airway of the trachea

Cell-gland secretes mucus

Fig. 43   The way the trachea works.

mental factors or specific disease organisms that attack the individual cells respiratory disease will follow. There are parallels between this system and protective mechanisms in the human respiratory system.

The bronchi enter the lungs and then divide and subdivide into a complex network of airways that are intimately associated, but not connected with, an equally complex network of minute blood vessels. It is here that the gaseous exchange of oxygen for carbon dioxide that is essential for life takes place. The lungs of the chicken are fundamentally different from those of mammals. The bird has no separate chest cavity or diaphragm and

the lungs are firmly attached to the wall of the chest and do not significantly expand and contract during respiration. Instead of being strictly 'in and out' organs acting like a bellows as they are in mammals where the air breathed in at each breath is almost completely breathed out before the next breath, the bird's lungs are 'through and through' organs. Inhaled air passes right through the lungs into a number of air sacs that completely line the bird's body cavity. In some species of bird they extend into the bones that are therefore hollow; this clearly reduces the weight of the bird and increases its flight potential. For instance, a large seagull with a wingspan of three feet only weighs 12oz.

The air sacs greatly increase the amount of fresh air available for the lungs to process and the air in them is recycled before being expired. The flexibility of this mechanism, linked with others in the circulatory system, explains the remarkable ability of some species of birds for sustained high energy activity and also the ability of some species to fly both at sea level and at very high altitudes, sometimes up to 20,000ft.

In the chicken the air sacs are vulnerable to infections picked up from the inspired air. They do not have complex linings like the trachea and bronchi and easily become infected. Unfortunately, if the bird has managed to recover from an acute respiratory disease and the infective agent has been removed from the trachea and lungs the air sacs often remain chronically infected, leading to relapses and illthrift in the bird. Postmortem examination shows thickening of the air-sac membranes and usually cheesy or purulent material in the air sacs themselves. This is a very significant feature in respiratory disease in poultry. The condition used to be described as chronic respiratory disease, as if it was a specific disease. It is however the end effect of a number of different primary conditions.

RESPIRATORY DISEASES

Respiratory disease is very common in chickens of all kinds and under all systems of management and its influence on the welfare of the birds and the economic success of all poultry enterprises cannot be overstated.

Localized Respiratory Disease

● Coryza.
Birds show only localized signs of disease with watery or purulent discharge from the eyes and beak. Affected birds look as though they have a 'cold'. Simple coryza is very infectious and is usually caused by bacteria. The condition often responds well to antibiotic treatment. It can be confused with the respiratory distress that is

caused by too much ammonia in the air in the house. In that case the stockman should be able to detect the ammonia and the birds usually also show pain and irritation of the eyes with the rapid development of blindness in some of the affected birds. Coryza may also be just one sign of a virus infection so once again an accurate diagnosis needs to be made.

● Pouch Breathing.
If the nostrils are blocked with mucus the sinuses under the eyes may puff in and out slightly at each breath. In severe cases the bird has to breathe with its beak open, like a person with catarrh.

● Sinusitis.
If the clinical signs of coryza are coupled with permanent swelling and inflammation of the sinuses under the eyes the condition is much more serious. In these cases there is often a watery exudate from the corner of the eye in addition to mucus at the beak. The cause may be mycoplasmal infection, or virus respiratory disease and an accurate diagnosis must always be made.

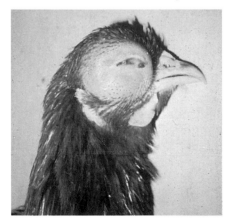

Fig. 44 Sinusitis.

● Swelling of the Head.
When this occurs in a number of birds in the flock it may be a sign of infection with

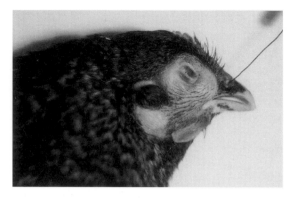

Fig. 45   Coryza showing blocked nostrils.

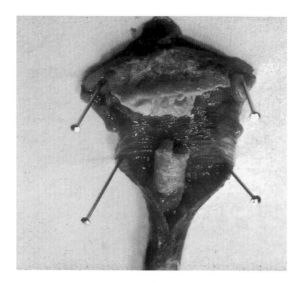

Fig. 46   Laryngo tracheitis. Blockage of trachea with exudate.

avian Rhinotracheitis virus, in which case some of the birds will clearly look ill and there will also be mortality.

● Laryngitis.
If the breathing is dry, laboured and gasping and the bird is clearly distressed at each breath the cause is disease of the larynx. If the condition occurs as a flock problem in birds of any type that are over 6 weeks old the cause may be infectious laryngo tracheitis that is caused by a virus. Coughing is a feature of this disease and if the affected bird coughs out bloody mucus this is the cause. There is usually mortality in the flock and the birds that die do so from asphyxia, caused by complete blockage of the windpipe with disease exudate. In these birds the comb and wattles of the dead birds are deep purple (cyanosed). Less severe cases also occur that, like most respiratory diseases, are not possible to diagnose accurately by observation alone. Fowl pox, some mouth infections and a very acute form of infectious bronchitis may all look very much the same and only veterinary diagnosis will differentiate them. Birds that recover from ILT remain as carriers of infection and a vaccination policy for the farm is usually necessary to prevent future oubreaks of the disease.

● Coughing is also seen occasionally in young birds that are being reared on long-established pure-breed farms where they have access to paddocks. The cause may be a parasitic worm, the gapeworm, that lives in the windpipe. The fungus infection Aspergillus also causes coughing in chronically affected birds.

Generalized Respiratory Infections

There are a number of specific infections, each of which can cause disease, but in practice there are often several factors that all contribute to a respiratory disease outbreak in a flock. The mix of factors greatly influences the severity of the outbreak but the symptoms in individual birds that the poultryman sees are very similar in all of them and it is often difficult to establish the primary cause. He should recognize the various symptoms but should not attempt to make a final diagnosis himself; there is so much overlap between the different diseases that this only causes confusion. To further complicate matters, some of the most important organisms causing respiratory disease, for example Newcastle disease, infectious bronchitis and avian influenza, occur in different strains that vary both in the severity and in the type of disease that they cause. The prevalence of these different strains of infectious agent also varies from year to year and the poultry vet must always keep up to date with the current situation in his region to help him to identify and control the different outbreaks with which he is confronted.

The specific organisms that can cause respiratory disease include:

● Infectious Bronchitis.
There are several different types of this virus and different variant strains occur in different years and in different locations. The vaccines available commercially do not give complete protection against all these strains and designing an effective vaccination programme for any particular farm is difficult. On problem farms this involves the necessity to carry out blood tests in depth in order to identify which strains of virus are present.

The clinical diseases that the different strains produce vary widely. All cause some degree of damage to the respiratory system but most also affect the reproductive system and have serious effects on egg production and egg quality. The respiratory lesions vary from a mild upper respiratory infection to severe tracheitis, bronchitis and pneumonia associated with airsacculitis.

● Avian Rhinotracheitis.
This virus is now widely established in chicken flocks of all kinds and often contributes to respiratory disease outbreaks. The clinical signs vary and include swelling of the head, tracheitis and bronchitis. Its presence in a flock must be confirmed by blood testing. Vaccination is an aid in the control of the disease but is of limited value on multi-age farms.

● Mycoplasma.
Mycoplasma gallisepticum, commonly known as MG, can cause acute respiratory disease characterized by coryza, sinusitis, bronchitis and airsacculitis. Its presence increases the susceptibility of birds of any age to other respiratory diseases and affected birds remain as continuous carriers of infection. Diagnosis is by blood testing and if found rigorous control measures must be started. Effective control of any disease involving mycoplasma is very difficult and must be carried out methodically under strict veterinary supervision in order to have any chance of permanent success.

● Newcastle disease, avian influenza, fowl cholera and E. coli can all cause generalized respiratory disease and are described in detail in separate sections later in this chapter

The severity of disease is influenced not only by the actual infectious agents but also by the age and type of bird, the state of its immune system and the environment in which it is kept. Post-mortem examinations and often follow-up blood tests are needed before a provisional diagnosis can be finalized. The veterinary investigation must be directed towards the identification of all the contributory factors, then in addition to setting up immediate treatment a plan can be made to prevent future outbreaks from occurring. In the absence of proper control many broiler farms have severe respiratory disease in each successive flock, particularly in the birds reared in the winter months between September and May.

In more generalized respiratory disease the birds' breathing may be coupled with wet gurgling sounds or partial sneezing, called snicking but when the lungs and air sacs are affected the clinical signs are not always obvious. Some of the birds will, however, look ill and breathing will be rapid. There will be a drop in food and water consumption and in egg-producing flocks clinical signs will soon be followed by a drop in egg production. If this is accompanied by the appearance of soft-shelled eggs or eggs with poor shells this may indicate a virus infection such as infectious bronchitis or Egg Drop Syndrome, but the possibility of Newcastle disease should always be considered. If there is concurrent infection with mycoplasma the symptoms will probably be more severe.

In the most severe forms of respiratory disease birds will stand around dejectedly with ruffled feathers and closed eyes and there will be high mortality. The disease may be caused by cholera, an acute strain of Newcastle disease or, rarely, avian influenza.

Most respiratory diseases in chickens can very quickly lead on to generalized E. coli infection, particularly in table birds where the stocking density is high and the ventilation and hygiene are of a poor standard. E. coli, like mycoplasma, makes an existing infection more severe and often causes high mortality.

NEWCASTLE DISEASE AND AVIAN INFLUENZA

(Fowl Pest and Fowl Plague)

For poultry farmers it is better to consider Newcastle disease and avian influenza together although they are caused by completely different viruses. Both can cause disease of widely varying severity, according to the strains of virus involved, as is the case with human influenza, and the possible symptoms shown in Newcastle disease overlap with those shown by influenza.

Influenza is primarily a respiratory disease but in severe outbreaks can cause almost 100 per cent mortality in a flock

in such a short time that respiratory symptoms in live birds do not have time to develop. Newcastle disease can also occur as a respiratory disease with very high mortality. The most recent outbreaks of this form of the disease were between 1970 and 1973 when there was a widespread epidemic in Europe that was of national importance to their poultry industries. In the very virulent outbreaks even baby chicks are fully susceptible and there is high mortality in them from pneumonia.

The disease also occurs in less severe forms involving diarrhoea, often stained green in colour, a drop in egg production in adult birds and, most importantly, nervous signs and behavioural changes in a proportion of the birds affected. A very mild form of the disease can also be caused by live vaccines that have become established on farms and cause infection in their own right.

Both Newcastle disease and avian influenza can be spread very quickly by air spread in birds that have respiratory symptoms, and via the droppings in all forms of the disease. Both diseases are potentially the most serious that can affect poultry and, additionally, avian influenza is so closely related to human influenza that there is always a risk of it causing disease in people. The recent (1997) outbreak of avian influenza in chickens in Hong Kong provides a good example of the serious public health implications of the disease.

For all these reasons it will be clear why for many years both diseases have been subject to legislation in countries with developed poultry industries. In Britain they were originally called Fowl Pest and Fowl Plague. They are classified as notifiable diseases under the 1981 Animal Health Act and anyone who suspects that a flock may be affected with either of the diseases must immediately notify either the State Veterinary Service within MAFF or the police. In practice the best procedure is for the poultry farmer to contact his own veterinary surgeon without delay so that he can carry out an immediate investigation and notify the State Veterinary Service only if he, with his special knowledge, thinks there is a possibility that either disease is present.

The diseases can occur in chickens of any age and the clinical signs of both diseases vary greatly. Any unexpected disease outbreak on a farm that occurs suddenly in a flock should be treated with suspicion by a poultry farmer and he should contact his vet for advice. It is impossible to generalize on the way the diseases may show in any new outbreak.

The nervous signs, particularly in older chickens, that are most suspicious are caused by brain damage and include a high-stepping gait, walking in circles, stargazing, abnormal pecking, abnormal positioning of the head and neck or complete inability to stand. A further complication in diagnosing Newcastle disease is that during an epidemic vaccinated birds sometimes become infected and show mild and indeterminate symptoms.

After a suspected case is notified to MAFF a visit will be made to the farm immediately by a state veterinary officer, who has the power under the legislation to take birds for post-mortem examination to confirm or negate a suspected diagnosis. If the case is confirmed by laboratory diagnosis the current government policy for control (which varies from time to time) will be applied. The farm and surrounding area will be declared an 'Infected Area' and movement of any poultry either within or out of that area will be strictly controlled. Measures to deal with the infected birds and to limit the spread of infection will be set up.

Control measures may include slaughter of infected and in-contact flocks in addition to strict hygiene measures to isolate individual farms and to control of all transport onto or from the affected farm. For Newcastle disease vaccination of all flocks in the surrounding area may be part of the policy, but there is no effective vaccine against influenza.

Outbreaks of influenza have usually been found to have been started by migrating waterfowl, many species of which can be permanent symptomless carriers of the infection and can spread it to domesticated chickens in their droppings. Once an infection becomes established in a chicken flock, spread to other flocks readily occurs.

Newcastle disease may also be introduced from wild birds, pigeons were responsible for a number of outbreaks based on Liverpool docks in 1983, but it is more frequently introduced by direct or indirect contact with infected poultry flocks. People and transport vehicles can also carry infection and spread it rapidly over long distances on contaminated clothing or farm dust on the vehicles. Tight hygiene precautions should be a part of routine management of all poultry farms in order to minimize the chances of introducing this dreaded disease.

Vaccination against Newcastle disease is very effective if it is carried out correctly and because of the unpredictable ways in which the disease can reach a farm all poultry farms should incorporate a vaccination programme into their management system. Table birds always pose particular problems with vaccination because they are often slaughtered before they have had time to develop full immunity.

CHOLERA

This is a very acute respiratory infection, usually affecting adult chickens, that is sometimes the cause of very high sudden mortality. It can affect commercial layer or breeder birds. Outbreaks are now uncommon in Britain, although the disease is still often seen in turkeys, but it is a common disease in some countries of the world where it causes serious economic loss.

The first sign that the poultryman sees is usually mortality, but when a detailed inspection is made a number of obviously sick birds will be seen. These tend to stand or lie round the walls of the house, or stand gloomily over the drinkers without actually drinking. An observant poultryman will also notice a distinctive smell in an affected flock.

The disease is caused by a bacterium, *Pasteurella multocida*. It can spread by direct contact between affected birds and also very commonly via the water that becomes contaminated with nasal exudate from birds as they drink or dip their beaks into the water, as sick birds often do. It also spreads in the droppings. These contain the bacterium in very large numbers because enteritis is associated with the condition. The bacteria can also live and multiply in mites, sparrows, rats, mice and other vermin and spread back to chickens from them. The disease is therefore most commonly seen in flocks where the standard of hygiene is poor and occurs most often during the autumn and winter months.

It responds well initially to antibiotic treatment but the environment remains infected and birds remain as carriers. Relapses therefore continue throughout the remainder of the flock's life so that continuous medication is usually necessary. Improving the hygiene on the farm is most important. Daily cleaning and disinfection of all drinkers and feeders should be a part of routine farm management and measures should always include control of vermin and possible intermediate hosts.

Unfortunately, commercial vaccine is only effective against some types of the disease. The vaccine is given by injection and two or sometimes three doses are needed. If disease is suspected in a vaccinated flock the vet should be contacted for advice.

Symptoms in an affected flock often suggest cholera to an experienced poultryman but diagnosis should always be confirmed by post-mortem examination and culture of the bacterium. Post-mortem lesions vary, but usually include large numbers of pinpoint haemorrhages (petechieae) in the internal organs, an enteritis with thick mucoid bloodstained material in the duodenum, and severe pneumonia with solidification of the lungs.

13 The Digestive System

STRUCTURE AND FUNCTION

The digestive system of the chicken is adapted to provide for the storage of food before it is digested, and also for the grinding up of coarse fibrous material.

The horny beak is designed to pick up food, so it must be hard and inflexible in chickens of all ages. In a healthy chick it is horny at hatching, and it is the action of the chick pecking through the shell (pipping) that enables it to hatch successfully. After hatching, it is important that the bones in the skull calcify quickly so that the beak is firmly anchored for effective pecking. Early virus infection or nutritional faults can delay this.

The beak leads into the cavity of the mouth that contains the small fairly rigid tongue. From the mouth, food material passes into the oesophagus and is prevented from passing down the windpipe and choking the bird by the larynx that acts as a valve and keeps the windpipe closed except when the bird breathes.

Food can then either pass directly into the stomach or can be retained in the crop for storage. The crop is a bag-like diverticulum of the oesophagus at the base of the neck. When space is available in the stomach the muscles of a healthy crop contract and pass the food on into the stomach for digestion.

The stomach is clearly divided into two portions. The first is the glandular stomach or proventriculus where food is mixed with digestive juices before passing into the muscular gizzard. The function of the muscular gizzard is to grind up food into a mulch that can then pass on into the intestine for further digestion. Sharp grit of suitable size is needed for this function. The grit also stimulates development of the gizzard muscle and in a healthy chicken a very strong effective grinding organ develops. In the gizzard, fibrous material such as grass stems and whole grain husks are broken down into a mulch so that they can be passed on together with the more easily digestible matter into the first part of the intestine, the duodenum that is a U-shaped tube. The U encloses the long, narrow pancreas that is a pale creamy pink colour and looks not unlike fat. One of its functions is to secrete enzymes that aid in protein and

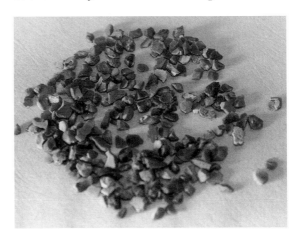

Fig. 47 Sharp hen grit.

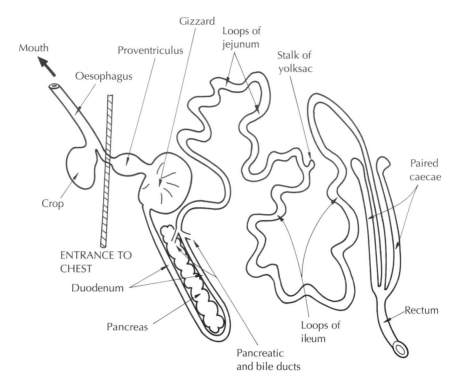

Fig. 48   The digestive tract

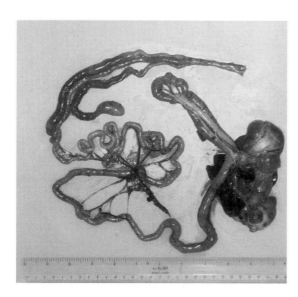

Fig. 49   The digestive system.

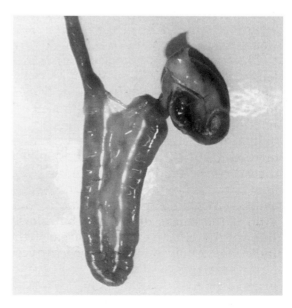

Fig. 50   The gizzard and duodenum
showing the pancreas.

fat digestion. These enzymes drain into the duodenum via three ducts and in some early virus infections of chicks these are damaged by the viruses. The pancreas cannot then function effectively and there is a resultant interference with digestion. This is part of the 'runting and stunting' picture. The pancreas also regulates glucose metabolism but this does not directly affect digestion.

The liver is a large roughly bilobed organ visible immediately the abdomen is opened. It is mahogany-coloured, except in birds that are very fat in which case it is a light yellowish brown. The liver is vital for many body functions but its digestive function is to produce bile. This is a bitter-tasting dark green fluid that can be stored in the gall bladder before discharging into the duodenum where it mixes with the food material and further aids in digestion. In some conditions excess bile is produced so that the birds droppings are green. This is a significant clinical sign in some diseases including certain forms of Newcastle disease. The small intestine continues as the loosely coiled jejunum and then, from the point where in the developing chick the yolksac was attached, as the ileum.

Digestion takes place along the whole length of the small intestine that has a tightly folded lining of digestive cells. The folds are prolonged into innumerable microscopic fingerlike projections called villi; this construction gives the chicken an enormous surface area across which digestion can take place. In runting and stunting disease of young chickens the causal viruses destroy the villae so that even if the chicks do not die but slowly recover the effective surface area of the intestine for digestion is much reduced and nutrients cannot be efficiently absorbed across it. This is the meaning of the term malabsorption. The result of this is that the chicks do not grow properly but remain runted and stunted.

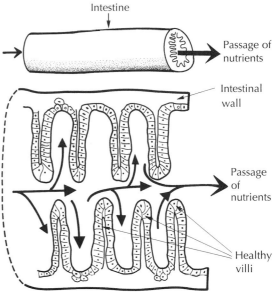

Shows the large area for the absorbtion of nutrients

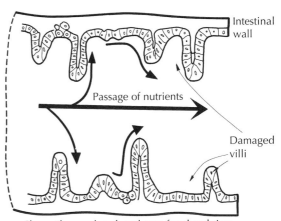

Shows the much reduced area for absorbtion

Fig. 51   Malabsorption.

At the end of the ileum is a four-way valve. The paired caeca start here as long blind-ending sacs that run backwards closely attached to the ileum that continues as the rectum. Some of the partly digested food passes by muscular action back from the ileum into the caeca where further fermentative digestion takes place. Material from both the ileum and caeca ultimately pass along the short

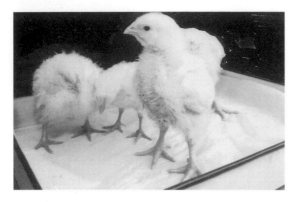

Fig. 52 Runting and stunting. Showing great variation in size of chicks by the time they are two weeks old.

rectum, usually separately, to be passed as droppings at the vent. Just inside the vent the intestinal canal is joined by the ureters, the urinary tubes from the kidneys. The reproductive tract also joins the rectum at the cloaca so the vent provides a common orifice for digestive, urinary and reproductive material.

There are therefore three quite different types of material that make up the bird's droppings and, additionally, eggs, sperm or any abnormal reproductive discharges also pass out at the vent. In the healthy chicken the droppings consisting of material that has travelled directly from the ileum are grey-brown, solid and fairly fibrous, those that have been excreted from the caeca are sticky and a much brighter brown, and those from the ureters (the bird's urine) are chalky white and semi-solid and are often passed with other droppings. Different diseases affect all these types of droppings in different ways according to the location of the disease problem, and careful examination of the nature of the droppings is a most valuable aid in accurate diagnosis.

DISEASES OF THE DIGESTIVE SYSTEM

Abnormalities of the Beak

Some deformities of the beak are of genetic origin and nutritional deficiencies will also lead to abnormal development. Most abnormalities are, however, the result of faulty beak trimming or of a management system that does not allow the bird to peck normally and keep its beak sharp.

The Mouth

Chickens with disease affecting this region are unable to swallow food normally and often stand around with their beaks partly open. Sometimes there is gasping breathing and there may be ulcers or scabs extending from the corners of the beak or on the tongue. The problem may be caused, both in baby chicks and broilers, by giving them food that is too finely powdered and low in fibre. This cakes when mixed with water, sticks in the mouth and cannot be swallowed. It soon becomes sour and infected and the condition is easily confused with a genuine infection of the mouth or with disease of the crop. Specific infections of the mouth include fowlpox, canker (trichomonas), staphylococcus or fungal infection. The exudates from these diseases quickly become foul-smelling and caked stale food accumulates at the back of the mouth. A laboratory diagnosis of these conditions is necessary.

The Crop

Regurgitation of sour food often indicates paralysis of the crop. The dilated crop appears as a pendulous bag that can be seen hanging down from the base of the neck. The cause can be Mareks disease, fungus infection or a nutritional fault. The crop also becomes paralysed if it is over distended or impacted with fibrous material. This may occur in chickens that are on a restricted feeding programme if the interval between feeds is too long. The condition was common in broiler breeders that were only fed on alternate days, called skip-a-day feeding. At feeding time the chickens were excessively hungry and ate too much too quickly, over-distending the crop. The condition is more likely to occur in birds that have not been given grit and have poorly developed gizzards, when the food retained in the crop quickly ferments and the dilatation become chronic.

The Stomach

The poultryman cannot recognize abnormalities of the stomach clinically but some are associated with dilatation of the crop. All cause some failure in digestion and affected birds of any age become unthrifty.

● Impaction of the Gizzard.
This is an important condition for all poultrymen to understand. The gizzard becomes full of a tightly constricted ball of fibrous material that also plugs the first part of the duodenum and prevents the passage of food, and even sometimes of water, so that the affected bird progressively starves to death. The impaction occurs most commonly with stemmy grass, straw or hay.

If birds of any age that have not had grit are transferred to free range where they have sudden access to stemmy grass, or if they are bedded on straw or hay, or hay is put in their nesting boxes, they will consume these materials and some will suffer from impaction. Later, food builds up in the crop, causing dilatation and often regurgitation. In badly managed flocks this condition can kill as many as 20 per cent of the birds.

Grit is seldom given to commercial broiler chickens that are on intensive management and are killed before they are seven weeks old. These birds are fed on a high-density low-fibre diet and the function of the gizzard to macerate fibrous material is not required. The gizzard muscles remain very weak in birds that have not been given grit; the gizzard remains small and digestion is potentially less efficient. In all birds kept on more natural extensive systems, and for chickens kept on as roasters to a heavy weight and finished traditionally on range or in barns grit is essential. If these birds have not developed a fully functional gizzard, deaths and illthrift from impaction are common. The condition can even be seen in broilers and very young replacement pullets where disease or bad management has led them to peck at their wood shavings litter.

Treatment of individual birds by opening the crop, removing the impacted material and stitching up again is unfortunately seldom successful as the basic impaction is usually in the stomach, out of reach of the surgeon. By adopting a rearing programme that includes grit of the right size from an early age, and introducing the birds to fibrous material for the first time with care, this condition can be largely prevented. Initial strimming of ryegrass paddocks, or grazing with sheep, are good management practices and straw used for litter should be carefully checked to make certain that it does not contain long palatable grass and weed fibres.

● Tumours.
Cancer of the stomach can occur in birds of almost any age. The commonest cause is Mareks disease.

● Newcastle Disease.
The glandular stomach (proventriculus) is affected in some cases of Newcastle disease. At post-mortem haemorrhages, inflammation and oedema are present. If these abnormalities are found a detailed flock investigation is necessary.

● Gizzard Erosion.

This is a specific disease in which the lining of the gizzard becomes ulcerated. It is most common in young birds and is usually caused by certain types of fish-meal being fed. There is sometimes quite severe haemorrhage into the gizzard and in all cases affected birds lose condition.

ENTERITIS

Enteritis is the general term for an inflammation of any part of the intestine, from the duodenum to the vent.

In baby chicks less than two weeks old it often causes very serious disease and high mortality. Virus infections, E. coli, salmonella and other bacteria are all possible causes.

In older birds there may be high mortality and living birds may look ill, huddling together with ruffled feathers. There may be staining of the feathers round the vent or even blockage and caking of the vent with droppings. In mild cases of salt poisoning or coccidiosis the birds are more thirsty than normal to compensate for the fluid they are losing in the loose droppings, and water consumption of the flock will rise. In cases where the birds look ill, however, water consumption and food intake all fall.

A poultryman can usually suspect that there is an enteritis problem of some kind in his flock from the appearance of the droppings and the condition of the litter in addition to clinical signs of disease. A final specific diagnosis, however, as with most diseases, will require laboratory tests and probably post-mortem examinations. In the serious infection where there is mortality these examinations do not present a problem but in the mild outbreaks there is often no significant mortality although serious infections such as salmonella or parasitic infestations may be present. In these cases it is almost always most satisfactory to sacrifice a number of birds so that a full post-mortem can be carried out and an accurate diagnosis made.

When there is severe diarrhoea the litter will become wet and this often makes the ventilation of the house inadequate so that it becomes humid and stuffy. Ammonia may also build up. If the droppings are sticky and glutinous they adhere to the surface of the litter and stop it 'working'. In either situation the chickens quickly become damp and bedraggled, the infection spreads rapidly and respiratory disease often follows and complicates the disease picture.

Parasitic infection or chronic coccidiosis may be the cause of enteritis in older growing birds or adults. Droppings and litter samples will initially be required by the vet, who will advise on what samples are needed to confirm a diagnosis.

Avian tuberculosis causes a persistent diarrhoea, coupled with poor production and progressive emaciation, usually in adult birds over a year old. This condition is seen in traditional free-range and farmyard flocks.

Droppings

An assessment of the type of abnormal droppings in any outbreak of digestive disease is a great help in establishing a diagnosis. First the type of droppings being examined must be established. Are they intestinal, caecal, urinary or an abnormal discharge from the reproductive system? Poultrymen often confuse the watery urine produced in some kidney diseases such as Gumboro disease with diarrhoea but this material is watery, often mucoid, contains white streaks of urate and has an unpleasant ammoniacal smell. In serious diseases of the reproductive system in hens, soft-shelled eggs can be confused with droppings if they have fallen under the perches where the hens roost and been broken or trampled.

Droppings from the digestive system may be:

Consistency
- Thin and watery.
  Diarrhoea is the most common sign of digestive disturbance that is noticed by the poultryman. Almost any intestinal disease can show as diarrhoea but simple factors to consider include an excess of salt in the ration, plant poisoning or simple indigestion from a change of food. If these are not the obvious reason for the problem infection must immediately be suspected.
- Sticky.
  This usually indicates infection, possibly with coccidiosis.
- Bubbly.
  Often seen in growing birds and may indicate virus infection.
- Foul-smelling.
  Usually indicates infection.
- Mucoid.
  May indicate parasitic infection but is a warning sign of many types of chronic digestive disturbance.
- Worms.
  Sometimes whole worms are excreted in the droppings.
- Blood.
  This is usually a sign of coccidiosis but can easily be confused with bleeding from the vent.
- Undigested food.
  Droppings may be abnormally fatty and greasy. In broilers this may indicate metabolic disease, for example Fatty Liver Kidney Syndrome. They may also contain obviously undigested food. In young birds this is usually an indication of malabsorption and the cause should be established. It may be virus runting and stunting. In older birds it

may be a sign that there is inadequate grit in the gizzards.
- Hard droppings.
  Hard dry droppings are seldom seen as a flock problem unless there has been a serious shortage of water but the condition is sometimes seen in individual birds and usually indicates terminal disease of some kind.

Colour
A change from the normal colour of droppings also indicates to a good poultryman that there may be a digestive problem of some kind.

- Dirty water-coloured.
  This clearly indicates a very acute diarrhoea.
- Cream-coloured.
  This may be caused by poor digestion of fat. It usually indicates a serious problem that needs to be identified.
- Mustard-coloured to dark brown.
  A sudden change within this normal range of colours may be an early warning of a problem.
- Green.
  This is caused by the presence of bile. This may indicate liver disease, stress or kidney failure. It is also present as a characteristic symptom in some types of Newcastle disease. It is therefore particularly important for the poultryman to establish the exact cause for the condition.
- Tarry.
  This indicates blood. It is present in birds with coccidiosis and in some other severe types of enteritis. It is easily confused with clotted blood from injuries to the vent.
- Blood-coloured.
  If there is frank blood in the droppings it usually indicates coccidiosis. This is always a serious condition and an accurate diagnosis must be established.

103

Causes of Enteritis

It will be clear that there are a large number of conditions in chickens that cause some type of enteritis. A good poultryman should be able to recognize the appearance of a problem quickly. He will then attempt to relate it to management, environment, nutrition or infection. More specific diagnosis will require the assistance of the veterinary surgeon and back-up laboratory examinations. Some infections causing enteritis include:

Viral Infections
- Infections causing malabsorption in young chicks, the runting and stunting viruses.
- Newcastle disease.
- Other enteric viruses.
  There are a number of viruses which are able to cause mild symptoms of enteritis in birds of all ages particularly on multi-age farms. Specific diagnosis needs in-depth laboratory investigations and is often not economically cost-effective.

Bacterial Infections
- E. coli.
- Salmonella.
  Usually only chickens less than four weeks old show severe clinical signs of disease but older birds can occasionally also show signs of infection and birds of any age can be carriers.
- Campylobacter.
  This common infection seldom causes severe clinical signs but is associated with a liver condition in adult birds.
- Spirochaetes.
  Diarrhoea associated with these bacteria is occasionally found in free-range flocks.
- Coccidia.
  This important group of protozoal parasites are described in Ch. 21.

- Tuberculosis.
  Causes chronic progressive emaciation with diarrhoea, usually in older birds.
- Parasitic Worms.
  Heavy infestation can cause illthrift and enteritis and the different conditions are described in Ch. 21.
- Necrotic enteritis.
  This is an infection that is important both in broiler chickens and laying hens. It shows as sudden mortality in a flock, often in birds in good condition, without any obvious symptoms being seen in the flock by the poultryman. A low-grade coccidiosis infection is quite often present in affected flocks. On post-mortem examination the small intestine from the duodenum to the ileum is thickened. The lining is grey and easily separates from the underlying tissue. The appearance of the intestine can easily be confused with coccidiosis but a laboratory examination will quickly establish that necrotic enteritis is a bacterial condition associated with the presence of clostridia. The condition is most common in birds that are kept under poor conditions of hygiene.

The After-Effects of Enteritis

After some types of enteritis the chickens return to normal very quickly. In others, for example salmonella, some birds may appear to be normal but may remain as carriers of infection. In these cases they can spread infection back to other birds and onto their eggs and are therefore a public health risk. In some young birds that suffer from severe enteritis caused by a malabsorption virus there is permanent damage to the intestine and the birds remain unthrifty.

Control

As with all diseases correct treatment should always be recommended by the vet.

Specific drugs to kill the various infections will of course be used, but often more importantly, these will be supplemented by treatment to aid digestion and replace minerals, vitamins or fluid and management changes to reduce the likelihood of future cases occurring on the farm.

DISEASES OF THE LIVER

A poultry farmer will not recognize liver disease in his flock, it will only be diagnosed at post-mortem examination.

- Fatty liver and kidney syndrome.
  This occurs in broilers between two and three weeks old that are growing well. It causes unexpected mortality. The cause is related to nutrition and is described in Ch. 9.
- Fatty degeneration of the liver in hens.
  Sudden death from this cause occurs in hens that are too fat. On post-mortem the liver is greasy and a pale yellowish cream colour. There is often severe haemorrhage from it or smaller haemorrhages within the liver tissue itself but in some birds no haemorrhages are present. Nutritional faults can cause this condition. See Ch. 9.
- Inclusion body hepatitis.
  This is a liver disease seen in young chickens, often pullets that are being reared for egg production, when they are between one and two months old. Mortality rises in an affected flock and at post-mortem examination the liver is found to be swollen and to have a typical microscopic appearance on which the veterinary pathologist can confirm a diagnosis. The cause is a virus but the disease has to be precipitated by the presence of Gumboro disease in the flock and has become much less common since vaccination against Gumboro disease has been normal practice.

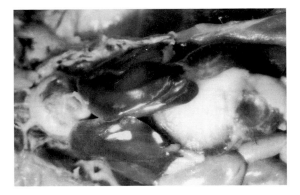

Fig. 53a   A liver of normal size.

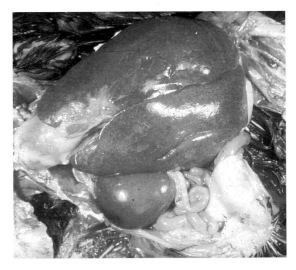

Fig. 53b   A liver affected with Big Liver Disease.

- Spotty liver disease.
  This is another condition that causes sudden death in young hens in lay. It is thought to be caused by the bacterium *campylobacter* that is widely distributed in farm environments but the disease is only seen in birds on free range and unidentified precipitating factors are probably associated with the development of the clinical disease. In a flock the disease shows as a sudden rise in mortality in birds in good condition. Birds that die have numerous

105

small pale brown spots (necrotic foci) in the liver. After a diagnosis has been made treatment with a suitable antibiotic normally shortens the course of an outbreak.

- Tumours.
  Several different types of tumour occur in the liver. The most common are caused by Mareks disease or lymphoid leucosis.
- E. coli, salmonella, poisons and many other conditions also affect the liver of chickens of different ages but their presence will not be detected unless a post-mortem examination is carried out.

SALMONELLA IN CHICKENS

Salmonella infections are important both because of the diseases that the different types can cause in the chickens and also because some of these infections can cause food poisoning in people who eat poultry products derived from infected birds. They are therefore of public health importance and are subject to controls under Food Hygiene and Safety of Foods Legislation.

Some strains of salmonella can be present in the ovary and reproductive tract of adult hens without causing serious clinical signs of disease or stopping the hens from laying eggs. These salmonella bacteria can then infect some of the eggs produced by these carrier birds.

In the 1980s the British Government found that salmonella infection in eggs was more widespread than had previously been thought. It was also established that a high percentage of eggs and egg products such as mayonnaise and bakers' products were not cooked before being eaten and that others, including soft-boiled and poached eggs were not heated to a high enough temperature to kill any salmonella bacteria present in them. This all caused the now famous Edwina Currie egg scare and in 1989 legislation was introduced, The Testing of Flocks Order, amid much publicity in the media in order to control salmonella infection in eggs. All egg producers were subjected to stringent periodic testing of their egg-producing flocks and flocks in which infected birds were found were slaughtered.

Salmonella can equally infect pure breeds, pullets being reared for commercial egg production and table birds of all kinds. In 1989 infection was actually more prevalent in broiler chickens than it was in commercial egg producers but table bird producers were not affected by the same legislation.

In addition to the spread from generation to generation that is possible with some strains of salmonella, rats, mice, sparrows and other vermin frequently carry infection. Once present on a poultry farm any type of salmonella is very difficult to eliminate because the bacteria can remain alive either on their own or within an intermediate host for long periods of time.

In the past salmonella was often present in commercial feeding stuffs but recent legislation passed as the Processed Animal Protein Order has led to a great reduction in feed contaminated with salmonella.

In 1992 all poultry farmers who produced products of any kind for sale for human consumption had to register under the Food Safety Act. This includes not only large commercial broiler farms but farm shops, small retailers and small poultry producers with bed and breakfast accommodation for visitors. The legislation makes all farmers and producers responsible for taking 'due diligence' in the production of their product to ensure that it is fit for human consumption. In practice this means that if a case of human food poisoning is traced back to a product produced by a particular poultry farmer the farmer, to avoid prosecution, must be able to prove that he took all reasonable measures to ensure the safety of the food for human consumption. This includes an ongoing policy for salmonella control on the farm.

All poultry farmers must therefore consider hygiene and disease control programmes, the keeping of flock records and routine testing for the absence of salmonella when designing the policy for managing their farm. Liaison between the poultry farmer and his vet will help him in this. It is not realistic for food producers to complain that recent food hygiene regulations are unnecessary; the public demand increasingly high standards for the food they eat and it is they who buy the poultry products. This public demand provides a real opportunity for the niche producers of quality poultry products to expand their market and profits but it progressively isolates the producers of poor quality, unhygienic poultry products.

Salmonella in Chicks

If the parent breeder flock is infected with salmonella there is a higher than normal mortality in the chicks both from yolk sac and general infection from the time of hatching. If the hatchery records are examined it will probably be found that the percentage of chicks that hatched normally was also lower than normal. This is because some of the embryos die from Salmonella infection during development.

If salmonella infection is picked up by the chicks on the farm after hatching, illness and deaths will start a little later, probably when the chicks are about three days old just at the age when normal early mortality in a healthy flock should be tailing off. On post-mortem examination of chicks less than a week old salmonella shows as yolk sac infection, infection of the navel, disease in the hips or general

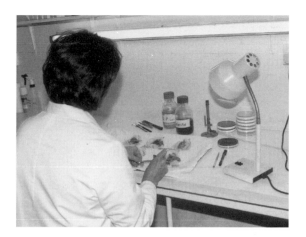

Fig. 54   Testing chicks for salmonella.

infection. There is also enteritis, often with diarrhoea and caking of the vent.

One type of salmonella, *Salmonella pullorum*, that spreads to chicks from the parent breeders does not produce disease in man but can cause very severe illness with white diarrhoea and mortality in baby chicks. This conditionthat was formerly called Bacillary White Diarrhoea, caused such disruption within the poultry industry in the first half of the century that the government introduced control policies. Blood testing of all breeder birds was carried out and birds that were found to be infected were slaughtered. In Britain the disease was almost eliminated by these measures by 1970 and government-control measures were relaxed. During the past few years, however, poultry veterinary surgeons have seen the organism more frequently again in pure collections, small domestic flocks of chickens and game birds. It may become progressively more serious in the future if control measures against the whole range of salmonella organisms affecting poultry are not conscientiously implemented by all poultry farmers.

Freedom of the whole flock from *Salmonella pullorum* has to be certified

107

for birds or eggs that are exported, and for birds going to some registered shows. There is a Government Poultry Health Scheme that enables flocks to comply with these requirements.

In all cases of unacceptable early mortality in chicks the vet should be consulted. It is important that, if salmonella is present in a flock, an accurate diagnosis is made without delay so that a policy can be drawn up that not only reduces the disease and subsequent illthrift in the affected flock but safeguards human health when the chickens are later slaughtered for human consumption. Also, by early diagnosis, infection can often be traced back to the parent breeder flock and action taken to control infection in it.

In untreated flocks, deaths from salmonella usually cease within 14 days but diarrhoea and illthrift often persist for another two weeks in some birds and in commercial broiler flocks the overall performance of an infected flock is usually reduced. In any case a percentage of surviving birds is likely to remain as carriers. Pullets can remain infected for months and table birds can still be infected at slaughter. In the processing plant these birds are not only a threat to human health individually but can cross-infect equipment and other carcasses which greatly increases the risk of infection in people eating poultry products produced at the slaughterhouse.

Salmonella in Hens

Adult birds carrying salmonella infections that can cause food poisoning do not show any clearly recognizable signs. Most of the birds appear clinically normal although some may show diarrhoea and illthrift, egg production may be lower than normal and mortality, particularly from egg peritonitis, may be higher than in a healthy flock. In breeder birds the hatchability of the eggs will be reduced and early mor-

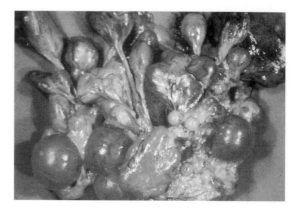

Fig. 55 A hen's ovary infected with salmonella (note some follicles on stalks).

tality and illthrift in chicks that do hatch will be high.

For the types of salmonella able to cause food poisoning the Salmonella Testing of Flocks Order 1989, and subsequent amendments, lays down a programme of swab testing for breeder flocks and pullets that are being reared for commercial egg production to check the absence of salmonella in them. Also, under the Zoonosis Order any salmonella isolations that are made by a laboratory from chickens at any time must be reported to MAFF. If it is thought necessary a state veterinary officer will then visit the affected farm to ensure that there is not an ongoing risk to public health and to make recommendations for future control of salmonella on the farm. Unfortunately in Britain this has become necessary more often recently because of the increase in the incidence of *Salmonella typhimurium* type 104, an increasingly common cause of human food poisoning.

Control of Salmonella
Treatment of flocks of any age is usually very successful if the right drug has been prescribed, but although antibiotic treatment advised by the vet on the basis of his laboratory diagnosis is often necessary for the immediate control of clinical

illness, long-term control measures should not be based on the necessity for treatment with drugs. Even after treatment a proportion of the birds often remain as carriers of infection and these can cause a risk to public health. A further cause for concern is that after treatment, remaining salmonella are likely to be resistant to the drug that was first used to control the infection in the flock.

Long-term control measures for salmonella should be based on:

- Hygiene.
  A comprehensive disinfection programme must be carried out when each poultry house is empty before it is restocked and routine measures should be taken to keep possible contamination of range paddocks as low as possible.

  Salmonella infections are very difficult to eliminate from farms because they can persist and multiply in wild birds, rats, mice and badgers. *Salmonella typhimurium* will rapidly colonize a variety of species that all provide a permanent reservoir of infection on the farm.
- Vaccination.
  An effective vaccine, given by injection, is now available against *Salmonella enteritidis*. A regular vaccination programme maintained on a farm will bring about a progressive reduction in the amount of infection with *Salmonella enteritidis* even on badly contaminated farms.

  All commercial breeder birds and pure breeds should be vaccinated during rearing as part of the overall control measures and the routine vaccination of all pullets that are being reared for commercial egg production should be considered. For small egg producers who rear their own pullets, the eggs can then be sold with a quality warranty that, increasingly in the

present-day market, enables them to command a higher price. A rapidly increasing number of supermarkets and other major purchasers of commercial eggs now sell eggs under quality trade marks that require that the eggs come from vaccinated birds. For example this applies to eggs sold under the Lion and the Freedom Foods designations.

Unfortunately there are not yet any vaccines against other salmonellae.
- Competitive Exclusion.
  This method of control involves giving a dose of a biological product that contains living 'useful' bacteria to all baby chicks immediately after hatching. The bacteria multiply and crowd out any later infection with salmonella or other harmful bacteria, preventing them from becoming established and causing disease. It is clearly also essential that the chicks receive the competitive exclusion product before they can become infected with salmonella. (Ch. 26)

Blood Testing of Breeder Flocks for Salmonella pullorum *Control*
Birds that are carrying *Salmonella pullorum* contain antibodies in their blood and these can be detected by a blood test.

- Swab Testing
  Regular swab testing of the environment in which the chickens are kept will detect the presence of Salmonella and, to some extent, the level of infection on a farm. This knowledge can then be used in designing a suitable hygiene programme for the farm.

E. COLI INFECTIONS (*ESCHERISCHIA COLI*)

E. coli is the name given to a large family of bacteria that are widely distributed in nature and are present in very large numbers in the digestive tract of all mammals and birds.

There are many different strains present in the environment. Some of them can cause serious disease in chickens in their own right; most of them only cause disease if there are predisposing factors that allow them to multiply in the tissues and cause general infection in the bird.

E. coli can infect almost any organ in the body and cause localized disease: arthritis, ear infection, infection in the reproductive tract, respiratory disease. However, it is most serious when it generalizes and causes an overwhelming infection that affects every part of the bird. This can occur in chickens of any age and E. coli septicaemia is one of the commonest diagnoses that a poultry vet makes in his day-to-day work.

The poultryman will not be able to make a definite diagnosis of E. coli infection because the clinical symptoms are not distinctive. In birds of any age diagnosis will be made by a post-mortem examination and it is not until an in-depth examination of every aspect of the flock's health and management is made that the factors contributing to the outbreak of disease can be identified. E. coli infections provide another example of the multifactorial nature of many diseases in poultry, and the importance of looking at all aspects of flock management and bird health, including vaccinations, when a disease outbreak is investigated.

In baby chicks E. coli can generalize from a yolksac infection or infection of the navel cord soon after hatching. The hip joints can also quickly become infected and the infection can become established in the bone marrow (osteomyelitis). E. coli can invade and multiply in the respiratory system if there are any predisposing factors or concurrent disease in the chicks, and then can generalize and cause high mortality with pneumonia.

In older chicks it can cause general infection if they are suffering from other diseases such as Gumboro disease or chicken anaemia virus, and at any age it can 'cash in' on a respiratory infection and cause general infection and mortality. If the environment for the chickens is poor, or if there are sudden changes in it due to weather conditions or thinning of flocks or movement to another farm, the associated stress factors often precipitate an outbreak of E. coli infection, there will be mortality and the diagnosis will be E. coli septicaemia.

In adult hens that have a reproductive failure that leads to eggs from the ovary being voided into the abdomen, the loose egg material quickly becomes infected with E. coli and causes septic egg peritonitis and death of the hen.

Laboratory examination will show what antibiotics can be used to treat a flock successfully but it cannot be over-emphasized that treatment with drugs is not the whole answer and in any E. coli outbreak a search should always be made to identify the underlying reasons for the disease.

TUBERCULOSIS IN CHICKENS

Avian tuberculosis occurs in many species of wild bird and also in pigs and rabbits. It only rarely, however, causes disease in man and is of little public health significance. In cattle it usually only infects individual glands but it interferes with clear results of a tuberculin test. For this reason alone it is important to eradicate the infection from poultry on all mixed farms. In chickens the disease spreads via infected droppings. The organism can remain alive in the soil or general environment for several years and once a traditional 'backyard' flock of chickens of varying ages becomes infected it is very difficult to eradicate the disease. Spread of infection

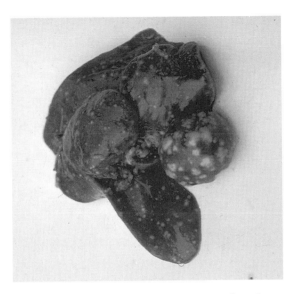

Fig. 57 Tuberculosis showing tubercles in the liver and spleen.

is usually slow and clinical disease is most common in birds over a year old except when the level of infection on the premises is very high because of poor hygiene and a heavily infected area over which the chickens range.

Tuberculosis causes a progressive wasting disease in chickens. Badly affected birds become emaciated and often have stained tail feathers because of persistent diarrhoea. In heavily infected flocks the percentage of infected birds is high enough to cause significantly poor egg production. However, the symptoms in life are not specific and can be confused with other diseases so diagnosis must be made by post-mortem examination. Liver, spleen and intestines show whitish nodules of various sizes. These are the tubercles, and in contrast to the rather similar nodules caused by cancers can often be squeezed out of the affected tissue like pips.

There is no treatment for affected birds and in a flock in which infection has been confirmed birds that are deteriorating in condition, and any others with persistent diarrhoea, should be destroyed. The flock should be moved into a clean building and onto fresh range and any further birds beginning to fall back in condition should be destroyed as soon as they are recognized. Clearly in a pure-breed flock, or a flock of 'pet' chickens where the birds have a sentimental value it is very difficult to eradicate the disease.

Young birds should not join an affected flock and, although it is not always possible, the aim should be to have a one-age flock until the infection has been eliminated. Ideally birds should be killed at the end of their first year's production during this control phase.

14 The Circulatory System

The circulatory system of the chicken is similar in principle to that of a mammal. There are refinements that allow for flight and other activities and the structure of the lung itself is different, but these variations do not affect a basic understanding of the blood flow in a bird.

Blood returns in the veins to the heart and enters the thin-walled right atrium and passes from there into the small right ventricle. The venous blood is pumped from there to the lungs where it picks up oxygen and gives up carbon dioxide. The oxygenated blood then returns to the heart in the pulmonary veins and enters the left atrium. It then passes into the strongly muscular left ventricle and from there is pumped all over the body,

supplying oxygen and other essential nutrients to the tissues. It then collects in veins again, having picked up carbon dioxide and other metabolic waste products. It returns to the heart, some of it via the liver and kidneys where toxic products are filtered from it, and enters the right atrium via the large vena cava.

CIRCULATORY DISEASES IN GROWING BIRDS

Failures of the circulatory system in young chickens are most frequently found in broilers and roasters. In these birds the very rapid growth puts a strain on the heart and lungs. Pullets reared for commercial egg production, which grow much more slowly, and also most young pure-breed birds are not so susceptible to circulatory diseases during rearing. Circulatory failures are most likely when chicks have not had the opportunity to exercise and develop their muscles during the first few weeks of life. It has now been firmly established that a shortage of oxygen in the tissues is associated with many of the circulatory diseases and cases of sudden death that are seen in chickens.

Flip-Overs in Young Table Birds

Very sudden deaths in apparently healthy birds start to occur in some flocks at any time after the birds are ten days old. The

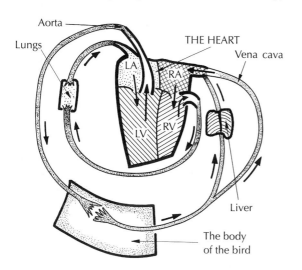

Fig. 58   The circulation in the chicken.

birds are found dead, usually on their backs. Sometimes a very brief period of convulsions is seen by the poultryman. In the industry the condition is called Flip-Overs. No infection is found on post-mortem examination and often the only abnormality is congestion of the carcass. Sometimes the liver is abnormally fatty. The cause is not fully established but the condition is thought to be a metabolic failure.

Roundheart Disease

This is also a condition of young birds. Affected birds are usually found dead from heart failure. In this condition the left ventricle is an abnormal shape, often very long, and not fully functional. The condition is commonest in some bloodlines of broiler chickens.

Broiler Dropsy

This is the commonest condition seen and may cause losses of over 20 per cent in some flocks.

From the time the chickens are three weeks old some birds in an affected flock will be seen to have swollen tense abdomens, to be less active than others in the flock and to be falling behind in condition. The developing combs are purplish in colour. Other birds are found dead and these too have very tense distended abdomens and a marked purple discoloration of all the exposed skin. New cases can continue to arise throughout the growth period of the flock and the condition is common in heavyweight roasters right up to the time they are due for slaughter. Post-mortem shows that the heart is poorly developed with very thin muscle. It is often grossly enlarged and dilated with venous blood. There is a variable amount of straw-coloured, often gelatinous, fluid in the abdomen and the lungs show congestion or oedema.

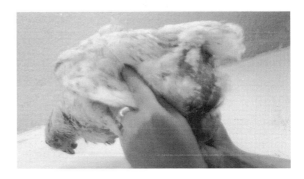

Fig. 59 A chicken with swollen abdomen typical of broiler dropsy.

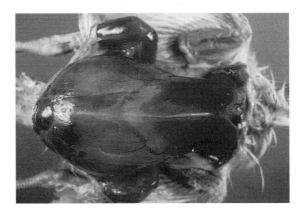

Fig. 60 Broiler dropsy.

When the efficiency of the lungs is reduced by a respiratory infection or when the quality of the air in a poultry house is poor because of the high stocking density and inadequate ventilation the uptake of oxygen in the lungs is less efficient and the bird suffers an oxygen deficiency. This is even more severe if the air in the house contains a lot of dust. Dust stimulates the production of mucus that acts as a barrier to air exchange and also introduces organisms that can cause respiratory disease. Oxygen deficiency is more severe if the poultry farm is at a high altitude where the air is less dense, for example in Mexico or parts of South Africa, and originally the condition was called Altitude Sickness.

113

The disease occurs in table birds kept under all systems of management. In birds in intensive broiler houses the quality of the environment is clearly of great importance. In birds kept on traditional farms wide temperature changes between daytime and night-time that commonly occur in the autumn and in the run-up to Christmas predispose the birds to the condition, particularly if they huddle together at night to keep warm. Sudden changes in weather conditions for birds in poorly ventilated draughty buildings will always increase the number of sudden deaths that occur.

CIRCULATORY FAILURE IN OLDER BIRDS

Heart Attacks

Heart attacks usually affect individual birds and are not serious flock problems unless severe stress factors, often associated with breeding, are operating. They are much more common in cockerels than hens, and are usually the result of sudden extra exertion, fighting or stress.

Most birds die suddenly and have very congested dark-coloured comb and wattles. Those that survive an attack remain very weak with obviously purple (cyanosed) comb and wattles and often gasping respiration. Some of these birds will recover slowly if put on their own in a comfortable pen and given old-fashioned tender loving care. Specific drugs to aid the circulation can also be useful.

Haemorrhage

In some birds of either sex sudden death occurs and the bird will be seen to be extremely pale. The cause is internal haemorrhage. In the cock this is usually from rupture of the aorta. In hens it is usually rupture of the liver. If it occurs in a number of hens in a flock the cause is probably nutritional and may relate to excessive fatness of the birds or to too much rapeseed being present in the feed.

Miscellaneous Conditions

Sudden death from circulatory failure can be caused by any condition that puts abnormal strain on the heart. These miscellaneous conditions become more common as birds get older and therefore are more often seen in pure-breed and backyard hobby flocks. Cancers of various kinds often cause death in this way in individual birds, often coupled with dropsy. Although the conditions are seldom significant in large commercial flocks, owners of pet chickens and hobby flocks can obtain a definite diagnosis in most cases if they submit the carcasses to their poultry veterinary surgeon. Sometimes such an examination reveals a hitherto unsuspected disease in the flock and remedial measures can be taken. The devil you know is often better than the devil you don't know.

Rat Poisons

Domestic animals are often poisoned by rat poisons containing warfarin but chickens are very resistant to this unless it is linked with other chemicals in potentiated Super Rat products. If poisoning occurs in a chicken, death is from internal haemorrhage coupled with the effects of the potentiating poison.

15 The Excretory System

STRUCTURE AND FUNCTION

The function of the kidneys is to remove nitrogenous and other waste products from the body so that the equilibrium of the body fluids is maintained under all circumstances. Good kidney function is essential for survival of the bird.

The urinary system consists of the paired kidneys, their ducts and the paired ureters that open into the cloaca at the vent.

The kidneys of the chicken are paired multi-lobed organs lying directly under the lumbar vertebrae, with which they are in contact, and covering the spinal nerves that combine into the sciatic nerve, the main nerve to the leg.

The waste material that forms the bird's urine is filtered into a network of excretory tubules in the kidneys and these unite into wider tubes that join to form a single ureter on each side. The ureters run posteriorly, parallel to the inner edge of the kidneys, to the cloaca. The normal urine of the chicken is white and semi-solid. It is usually passed with faecal material and forms part of the droppings of the bird.

The metabolic rate of birds is capable of wide variation and the amount of waste products that are produced as a result of the different bodily activities therefore also varies widely. For example there is only a short period of approximately a month between the time that a pullet of an egg-producing strain of chicken begins to mature, usually when she is about sixteen weeks old, and the time that she comes into full lay. During this time she is still growing, so she needs food for growth; her reproductive system is rapidly increasing in size and beginning to produce eggs so her protein metabolism becomes much more complex, and she begins to need extra calcium to provide the shell for each egg. Furthermore her behaviour changes as she starts nesting and, in breeder flocks, mating. All these activities increase her metabolic rate and result in the production of additional

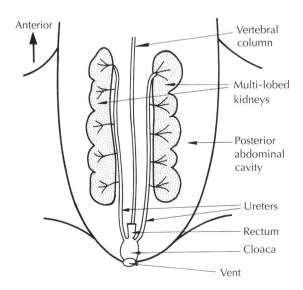

Fig. 61 The excretory system.

115

and often toxic waste products that must be efficiently excreted.

DISEASES OF THE URINARY SYSTEM

There are very few infections that specifically affect the urinary system and most of the cases that a poultry farmer will encounter will be from kidney failure.

Kidney Failure

The end effect of many diseases in chickens is kidney failure. Affected birds are dull and dehydrated. The feathers round the vent are often stained white and the birds may produce evil-smelling white liquid droppings that contain large amounts of urate. Some birds may have powdery chalky deposits on the comb and wattles, or have stiff joints. The feathers appear dull and lifeless and affected birds may stand near the drinkers as if they are thirsty. They do not eat and some may show nervous signs caused by the accumulation of toxins. These birds may have a high-stepping gait or convulsions. Kidney failure is usually very rapidly progressive and affected birds soon die.

Both the signs that a good poultryman will see in living birds and the post-mortem findings are fairly easy to recognize. It is important, however, that a diagnosis of kidney failure is always regarded as the start of an investigation and not the answer to it. The veterinary investigation must work back from the simple post-mortem findings to the primary cause of the problem if a useful contribution to the future health and progress of the flock is to be made.

Post-mortem findings:

- The kidneys are an abnormal colour and texture.
- The bird is dehydrated.
- There is often accumulation of urate in the kidney tubules and ureters.
- Often there are also chalky urate deposits on the heart, liver and other organs (visceral gout).

Some common causes of kidney failure:

- Stress.
- Poisons.
- Disease, particularly Gumboro disease in chicks.
- Absence or atrophy of one kidney.
- Excess calcium in the ration (young birds).
- Excess protein in the ration.
- Lack of water.
- Overheating.

Stones in the Ureters (Urolithiasis)

This condition occasionally occurs and causes sudden mortality in a young egg-producing flock as the birds approach peak production. There are no clinical signs that the poultryman can see. On post-mortem the kidneys show damage and the ureters are grossly distended with stones and gelatinous exudate. The cause is not fully understood but very high calcium in the ration before it is required for eggshell production, excessively high protein, shortage of water and infection with infectious bronchitis may all be implicated.

Tumours of the Kidney

These are usually caused by Mareks disease.

Chick Nephropathy

This term describes the death of a large number of chicks during the first three days of life from kidney failure. (See Ch. 24.)

16 The Nervous System

STRUCTURE AND FUNCTION

The nervous system of the chicken is in principle similar to that of mammals. It consists of a complex brain with associated cranial nerves, the spinal cord with nerves serving the wings, limbs and other regions of the body, and the much less obvious and more diffuse autonomic system of nerves whose function is to maintain an automatic control over the body and its functions.

For the study of disease it is convenient to divide the system loosely into three regions: the head and neck, the legs and wings, and the internal organs.

- The brain consists of the cerebrum, the cerebellum, small separately defined regions with highly specific functions, a core of spinal fluid that extends down the spinal cord, and a membranous covering, the meninges. Paired nerves from the brain go to the eyes and ears and nerves go to the beak that is very sensitive. Nervous impulses both leave the brain and reach it in the main spinal cord, located for protection within the vertebral column, and paired nerves from it service all parts of the chicken, the first series of nerves innervating the structures of the head and neck.
- The nerves from the wings unite into a complex plexus situated near to the shoulder joint before they join the spinal cord.

In the back region of the chicken, at the junction between the last free thoracic vertebrae and the synsacrum, there is a weakness in the vertebral column. In rapidly developing meat-type chickens this can lead to dislocation and paralysis. This condition is called kinky back. (See Ch. 11.)

The nerves for the legs emerge from the spinal cord along the posterior part of the vertebral column under the kidneys and unite into the thick sciatic nerves that go to the legs and feet. The spinal cord terminates in the sacral region that innervates the tail and the region round the vent.

- The nerves to the internal organs are provided by the autonomic nervous system. These nerves are very fine. They originate in spinal nerves and divide into a network that links all the internal organs with both the spinal cord and the brain.

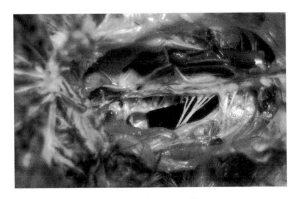

Fig. 62   Kidney and spinal nerves.

DISEASES THAT CAUSE NERVOUS SIGNS OR PARALYSIS

Disease of the brain itself shows as some type of change in the behaviour of the bird. This can vary from slight changes in temperament through convulsions to general paralysis or sudden death and are described in detail in the chapter on Signs of Ill Health (Ch. 6). Diseases of individual nerves will, on the other hand, show as more localized abnormalities relating directly to the region innervated. Examples are abnormal posture, lameness or partial paralysis. Disease of the autonomic system does not show in a distinctive manner; affected birds usually become progressively unthrifty and often have digestive problems.

There are only a small number of conditions that cause specific nervous signs in chickens and if the poultryman sees any problem involving signs of abnormal behaviour he must always consider the possibility of Newcastle disease first. Nervous symptoms are often not easy to spot in a flock if the birds have been suddenly disturbed. Normal behaviour overrides the abnormalities in all but the most severely affected birds. Individual birds or the whole flock should be examined when the birds are as relaxed as possible. When investigating a problem the vet should have an opportunity to look at live affected birds to supplement post-mortem examinations.

Nervous Conditions in Chicks Less than One Month Old

- Epidemic tremor (Avian Encephalomyelitis).
  This disease is caused by a virus that is transmitted from the parent breeders via the egg. Symptoms are usually first seen when the chicks are a few days old and are then shown by more chicks in an affected flock over the next few days. The affected birds are dull and reluctant to move, they cannot balance and they walk abnormally, also showing muscular weakness and collapse. A very rapid tremor develops in some affected birds and if this is found it distinguishes the disease from crazy chick disease. The tremor is best detected by placing an affected bird in the palm of the hand, when the vibration can be detected even if it cannot be seen. Alternatively a suspect bird may be put onto an enamel post-mortem tray, when the vibration often makes the tray rattle.

  There is no treatment for epidemic tremor. Affected birds should be destroyed on humane grounds. Surviving birds often remain very nervous and flighty and have to be treated with special care.
- Crazy Chick Disease.
  This is a nutritional disease caused by a deficiency in vitamin E. (Ch. 9)
  Chicks show a variety of nervous signs but no tremor.
- Aspergillus.
  The fungus infection that causes brooder pneumonia sometimes affects the brain and causes nervous signs and mortality in baby chicks less than three weeks old. The condition will only be diagnosed at post-mortem examination.
- Salmonella.
  Salmonella infections in young chicks occasionally involve the brain, in which case there are associated nervous signs. Diagnosis by post-mortem examination and culturing from the brain is necessary. The condition will probably be seen in only a few birds in a severely affected flock in which other birds show more typical symptoms.

Nervous Conditions in Older Birds

The specific conditions are described in more detail in the relevant chapters.

- Newcastle Disease.
  Any of the changes in behaviour caused by brain dysfunction may be shown in birds of any age.
- Other Virus Infections.
  Some other viruses can also affect the brain. Infectious bronchitis in some of its forms causes flightiness or sometimes aggression in an affected flock. Compulsive head shaking is also sometimes seen.
- Agricultural Chemicals.
  Clinical signs may be convulsions, tremors or paralysis.
- Poisoning with Anticoccidial Drugs.
  Ionophore poisoning causes paralysis.
- Botulism.
  This bacterial toxin causes paralysis.
- Mareks Disease.
  Mareks disease in one of its many forms may cause paralysis in chickens of any age over one month old. The virus causes infiltration of nerves with lymphoid cancer cells and these prevent proper functioning of the affected nerve.

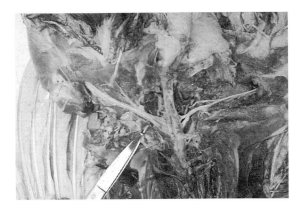

Fig. 63 Fowl Paralysis (Mareks disease). Sciatic nerve on one side is thicker.

If the nerve to the eye (optic nerve) is affected the bird will be blind.
- Ear Infections
  Loss of balance in individual birds in a flock may be the result of ear infection.
- Kidney Failure.
  In advanced cases of kidney failure the affected bird may show abnormal behaviour, for example a high-stepping gait or twitching. The cause is the build-up of toxins that have not been excreted by the damaged kidneys.

119

17   The Eye

STRUCTURE AND FUNCTION

The eye of the chicken is similar in principle to that of a mammal. Light first passes through the thin protective membrane at the front of the eye, the conjunctiva. This is adherent to the transparent anterior part of the eyeball itself, the cornea.

Light then passes through the aperture of the iris, the muscle that regulates the size of the pupil, then through the lens and onto the retina at the back of the eye. Here the light is recognized by specialized cells that transfer the information to the optic nerve that leads from the back of the eyeball directly to the brain.

The eye is protected by the upper and lower eyelids and there is also a small third eyelid situated at the inner corner of the eye.

Infectious organisms, dust particles and dirt are all picked up by the eye but there are two glands, the lachrymal and the Harderian glands, that lubricate it and produce tears that keep the region moist and wash debris away down the tear-duct to the back of the nasal cavity. These two glands have another important function, they are able to stimulate the bird's immunity to infections that reach the eye. Their ability to do this is utilized in the vaccination of chickens by the spray or eye-drop methods.

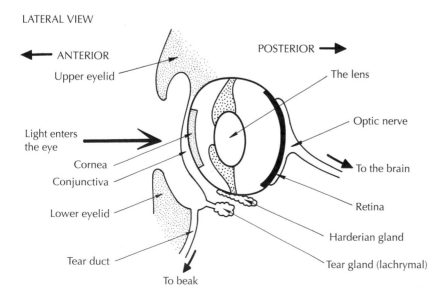

LATERAL VIEW

ANTERIOR

POSTERIOR

Upper eyelid

The lens

Optic nerve

Light enters the eye

To the brain

Cornea

Conjunctiva

Retina

Lower eyelid

Harderian gland

Tear duct

Tear gland (lachrymal)

To beak

Fig. 64   The structure of the eye. Lateral view.

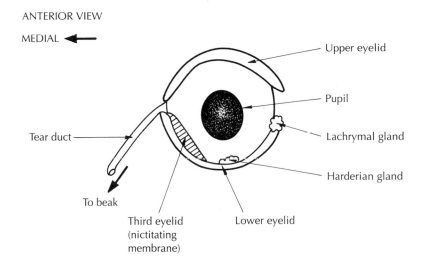

ANTERIOR VIEW

MEDIAL ◄——

Upper eyelid

Pupil

Tear duct

Lachrymal gland

Harderian gland

To beak

Third eyelid
(nictitating
membrane)

Lower eyelid

Fig. 65   The structure of the eye. Anterior view.

DISEASES OF THE EYE

The signs of eye disease that can be recognized by the poultryman can conveniently be divided into three sections.

Blindness

It will be the behaviour of an affected chicken that will draw attention to the condition. The bird will have difficulty in finding food and water. If it is a chick it will quickly lose condition and if it is an adult bird it will additionally probably seek solitude and skulk on its own away from the flock.

- The only significant cause in young chicks is a failure in the development of the retina. This is usually the result of absence of white light during the first few days after the chick hatches.
- Ammonia.
  In older birds excess ammonia in the air in the poultry house is almost always the cause of the problem if a significant number of birds are affected. This condition can be found in birds of any age kept on litter or in a laying house where droppings accumulate

under the floor of the house. Poor ventilation and damp conditions allow ammonia to build up. It first stimulates the tear gland and glands in the trachea, causing the birds to have runny eyes and bubbly breathing but the glands are rapidly destroyed so that both the eye and the trachea become dry. Inflammation of the conjunctiva and deep ulceration of the cornea rapidly follow. This always appears to cause the birds real pain and distress and presents a very typical picture to the poultryman. The birds rub their heads on the ground or scratch their faces. They stand around with ruffled feathers and eyes tightly shut. The birds do not eat and if handled, the eyelids go into spasm. Treatment of individual birds with soothing eye ointments is helpful but the damage to the eyes takes a very long time to repair, birds remain distressed and their condition deteriorates and the overall response to treatment is therefore usually slow.

- Mareks disease occasionally causes blindness in individual adult birds when a tumour involves the optic nerve.

121

Watery Discharge from the Eyes

This is a sign of respiratory disease. There may also be swelling of the sinuses under the eyes so that it is impossible for the birds to open them normally.

Inflammation of the Eyelids with Crusting or Bleeding

This may be the result of a respiratory infection if the exudate becomes infected with bacteria such as staphylococci or pseudomonas. Crusty lesions around the eye also occur in cases of fowlpox, in which case there are usually other scabby lesions on the face and diagnosis is not difficult. When the infection causes irritation, birds rub their heads along the ground or scratch their heads or eyes with their feet as they do in ammonia poisoning. New bacterial infection is introduced in this way and scabs develop. Inflammation with crusting or bleeding may also be the result of peck wounds in a flock where there is aggression.

If these localized conditions only occur in individual birds treatment with antibiotics and ointments is often successful. Affected birds must be put in a separate pen both to prevent further damage occurring and to limit the spread of infection to other birds.

18 The Ear ————————

The fowl has acute hearing. The entrance to each ear is a simple circular aperture on the lateral side of the head.

Specific disease of the ear is rare and the only condition recognized in individual birds in a flock is sepsis. The affected bird will suffer loss of balance and possibly convulsions. If there is infection of the ear canal, exudate can be seen. The cause is a bacterial infection, often with staphylococcus and treatment with antibiotic and ear lotion is often successful. In cases in which the middle or inner ear is affected there may be no exudate and a diagnosis from clinical signs cannot be made.

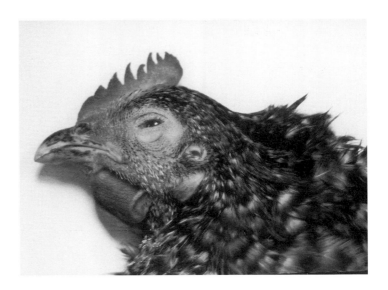

Fig. 66   The ear.

19 Mareks Disease and Tumours

MAREKS DISEASE

Mareks disease causes great loss to the chicken industry world-wide and is of concern to all poultry farmers. It is caused by a herpes virus and once a chicken becomes infected it remains so permanently and it can spread infection in its feather dust and dandruff intermittently for the whole of its life. The virus can also remain alive in the environment and capable of infecting new chickens for over a year so that, once a poultry farm has become infected, it is very difficult indeed to eradicate the disease.

The disease shows in a number of different ways. After the chicken picks up the infection the virus multiplies and during this stage the bird may look ill and may even be partially paralysed for a brief period as has recently been the case in some broiler chicken flocks where the affected birds have been named 'floppy chickens'. This condition started to occur in 1990 in flocks of broiler chickens about 35 days old in which a large number of birds in a flock suddenly became paralysed. The chickens recover spontaneously after 48 hours, but after recovering, a percentage of the birds in the flock develop typical Mareks disease tumours if they are kept on beyond the age of seven weeks.

In chickens that have contracted Mareks disease the way in which the disease develops varies according to the breed, sex and individual susceptibility of the chicken. After the initial phase that happens in all birds many of them will never show clinical signs at all. Some breeds and strains of chicken are more resistant than others and when buying pure breeds or unvaccinated commercial birds a poultry farmer should always enquire whether Mareks disease has been a serious problem on the vendor's farm. Some breeders have worked assiduously over a lifetime in order to develop resistant strains but others consistently suffer serious uncontrolled disease outbreaks. Before the first commercial vaccine was available the Sykes strain was particularly resistant.

In birds in which disease does show again it occurs in the form of a virus cancer, and this can also develop in different ways according to the individual susceptibility of the bird. In the most susceptible ones it causes rapidly growing tumours in almost any internal organ. The birds die quickly and tumours can be seen and diagnosis made on post-mortem examination. More slowly growing cancers also occur.

If the cancer cells invade nerves a number of clinical conditions may be recognized according to which nerves are involved. If the nerves to the legs or wings are affected the bird will show lameness, paralysis or drooping wings on one or both sides of the body. These are the classical signs of 'fowl paralysis' – the original name for Mareks disease. If a nerve to the head or neck is affected the bird may stand with a twisted neck, stargaze or walk in circles, in which case the signs are impossible to distinguish from Newcastle disease without laboratory tests. If the nerve to the eye is affected the bird becomes blind.

If nerves to the internal organs are affected there will be dysfunction and the bird will progressively lose condition and probably die, often from kidney failure. If the nerve to the crop is affected the crop will be unable to contract and will become distended with food that quickly ferments and becomes foul-smelling.

A careful post-mortem examination will show the affected nerves to be thickened and to have lost their normal structure. However, particularly where autonomic nerves are involved, these gross changes are very small and microscopical examination of stained lengths of affected nerves are necessary to confirm a diagnosis.

Mareks disease in any form makes birds more susceptible to other diseases because it reduces the efficiency of the immune system. Conversely, an outbreak of clinical Mareks disease in a flock carrying infection without showing any symptoms can be brought on by stress or by another disease affecting the flock. These are further examples of the multifactorial nature of many disease outbreaks in chickens and draw attention to the importance of a positive policy for disease control on a poultry farm so that the number of potential disease challenges to the birds is reduced. Some outbreaks of Mareks disease can be truly disastrous. Mortality of 80 per cent of all the birds reared is often reported in pure-breed flocks and 25 per cent mortality in susceptible commercial egg-producing flocks between the time the birds become sexually mature at about 16 weeks of age and about 30 weeks old, when they are at peak production, is common in unvaccinated birds.

A vaccine was developed in Britain in 1970 at the Houghton Poultry Research Institute and this, and vaccines developed later, have made control of the disease possible. However, under some circumstances vaccination is not completely effective and even vaccinated birds become clinically diseased. The vaccine should be given, preferably at day old, before the chickens can pick up infection. It acts, not by preventing subsequent infection but by stopping the infection from causing the clinical disease. In fact, it blocks the disease. Vaccinated chickens continue to carry the virus and they can also spread it to other birds in their feather dust and dandruff, so it is wise to consider all poultry farms with chickens on them to be infected, whether the birds are vaccinated or not.

The best vaccination programme for any particular farm should be decided by consultation with the farm vet and the vaccine manufacturer. Severely affected farms need to use a stronger vaccine and a second vaccination when the chicks are between two and three weeks old may be necessary. Vaccination has to be done by injection, and in day-old chicks bought commercially is carried out at the hatchery before the chicks are delivered to the farm. Pure-breed producers and small independent breeders of poultry must vaccinate their own stock and will require training and supervision before they can undertake this accurately themselves. The live Mareks vaccine is very fragile and has to be used within two hours of preparation and a complication for small breeders is that it is manufactured in minimum quantities of 250 doses. This means that each time a bottle is opened to vaccinate a small number of chicks much of the vaccine has to be wasted and the unit cost of the vaccine per chick actually vaccinated is therefore higher than in a large flock. Unfortunately this problem is typical of many that have to be faced by the smaller poultry farmers because the pharmaceutical industry is geared to the treatment of large numbers of birds in any single flock and the value of most individual chickens is low compared with other domestic animals or pets.

Some human cancers are caused by viruses and there are similarities between the ways in which some of them develop and Mareks disease. The research that has been carried out on every aspect of the disease in poultry has been of great benefit to the knowledge of human virus cancers.

OTHER TUMOURS

Poultry farmers with small flocks and pure-breed collections where the birds are kept until they are old are often concerned to know the reasons for unexpected deaths. If a post-mortem is carried out on these birds some of them may be found to have tumours or cancers of some kind. These occur more frequently with advancing age in chickens, as they do in other animals, and are not usually of economic importance. In commercial chickens during their first year in production most of the tumours now seen are caused by Mareks disease but in breeds in which control measures have not been taken to reduce the infection in the breeding flocks deaths from leucosis may occur. The diagnosis of tumours can only be made at post-mortem examination and the possible significance of any tumour found will have to be related to the history of the flock.

The Leucosis Group of Viruses

These cause tumours mainly in the liver and spleen of adult birds. The signs seen by a poultryman are not distinctive although when the tumours in the liver are very large the abdomen of a bird may be distended. This condition used to have the popular name of Big Liver Disease. Sometimes there is associated circulatory failure and the swollen abdomen is tense with dropsical fluid.

Leucosis viruses are egg-transmitted from one generation to the next and the susceptibility to them is related to the strain of the bird. Breeding programmes to eliminate the infections were started by commercial breeding companies a number of years ago and the disease is now rarely seen in commercial hybrids. It is found more frequently in individual pure-breed birds at post-mortem examination but even in these it is now not common. There is no treatment and vaccines have never been developed.

Other Cancers

Malignant tumours occur in individual adult birds of all strains. They most frequently affect the reproductive tract, the intestines and the various abdominal membranes, the peritoneum, the mesentery and the ovarian ligament. They are only of occasional commercial significance in some breeds of flocks. When they do occur no treatment is possible.

20 Diseases that Affect the Skin ——

Observant poultry farmers will quickly notice any abnormality affecting the skin of their birds. Some of these conditions only affect individual birds and some may not be true skin conditions but signs of other diseases. All, however, may be important indicators of the general health of a flock.

Swellings of the Head

- If the swelling is under the eyes or under the chin the cause is most commonly a respiratory infection.
- If the swelling affects the whole head it may be the result of infection with avian rhino-tracheitis virus. This can affect birds of all ages, will be a flock problem, and will be associated with obvious illness in a percentage of the birds.
- Similar swelling in individual adult birds may be the result of peck wounds that have become infected. The swelling may spread to the back of the neck. This condition is most common in breeder flocks in which the peck wounds are made by the cock at mating.

Abnormalities of the Comb and Wattles

- Scabby lesions may be the result of peck wounds, but fowl pox should always be considered, particularly in small pure-breed flocks in which birds are sent for show. In this disease that is now un-common, crusty pox lesions occur around the base of the beak and extend into the mouth, round the eyes and on the comb and wattles. Once pox virus is present in a flock it is very difficult to eradicate as it can remain alive outside the chicken for over a year. Rigorous hygiene measures are necessary to effect some control and a vaccination programme must be introduced.
- Favus.
  This is a fungus infection mainly affecting adult birds. The condition is rare except in pure breeds but it is contagious and should therefore be controlled. Small white areas first appear on the comb and wattles and slowly grow together until the whole area becomes hard, white and sometimes crusty. Anti-fungal ointments and thorough regular disinfection of the bird's accommodation, preferably with an iodine disinfectant, are often effective.

Diseases That Cause Slimy Skin

There are two rather similar skin conditions that occur in both broilers and pullets at any age between three and ten weeks. A number of birds in the flock are seen in which a wing or a thigh appears moist and shiny. Birds in affected flocks are usually not growing well and have become uneven with rising mortality and if the birds that die are not collected from the house very soon after death the carcasses putrefy rapidly. Any live birds that

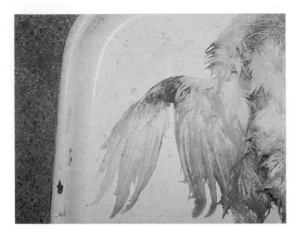

Fig. 67 Gangrenous dermatitis, showing wet loose feathers.

show signs of the disease quickly become ill and die. On examination it will be seen that some of the feathers have fallen out and the skin is slimy and sloughs away when rubbed with a finger.

These conditions are gangrenous dermatitis and blue wing and they follow infection with either Gumboro disease or chicken anaemia virus. These diseases affect the immune system and allow bac-teria present in the environment of the poultry house to infect the chickens and cause gangrene. Clostridia and staphylo-cocci are the main species involved and these are particularly common on dirty farms; good hygiene reduces the incidence of the diseases.

Treatment of affected flocks with antibiotic may be useful but should always be combined with measures to improve the general health of an affected flock. Policies to prevent the underlying infections in future flocks reared on the farm and attention to hygiene are most important. These conditions are further examples of multifactorial diseases in chickens.

Skin Tumours

Mareks disease can occasionally cause tumours in the skin.

Scaly Leg

Thickening and scaliness of the legs may be caused by a mite and is described in Ch. 21.

21 Parasites —————————

INTERNAL PARASITES

Parasitic worms and coccidia are the only two groups of internal parasite that commonly cause disease in chickens in Britain.

Chickens on free range can also act as carriers for the blackhead parasite, Histomonas, that causes severe disease in turkeys and gamebirds. It is rare for chickens to become ill with this disease but it is important for poultry farmers to be aware of it because the chickens can spread it to turkeys. This is one of the reasons why, before effective drugs for its control were available, farmers were always advised to avoid keeping turkeys and chickens together.

The various parasites are described in some detail because they are of particular importance to all poultry farmers who keep their flocks under traditional range or barn conditions, and also to pure-breed poultry farms and to breeders of replacement pullets. On many of these farms there is continuous stocking of both paddocks and poultry houses which enables the parasites to become established.

Intestinal Worms

The Large Roundworm (Ascaridia)
This worm is present on most rearing and laying farms. It can be present both in flocks on litter and on free range.

The worms are white in colour, fairly stiff and rigid, and up to about three inches long. They are present in the small intestine and the eggs pass out in the droppings. The eggs have thick, resistant, sticky outer coats that make them very difficult to wash off walls and floors during the farm cleaning programme and they can remain alive for over a year. On range the eggs can also be swallowed by earthworms and other invertebrates and transferred in this way to new chickens if they eat the earthworms. The worm is also commonly found in a variety of wild birds including starlings, blackbirds and thrushes, magpies and other crows and these birds can infect paddocks when they pass droppings on them. On a poultry farm infection is particularly likely to build up round feeders if the birds are fed on range and also under trees in the paddocks in which wild birds roost.

The worms develop in the chicken and take 6–8 weeks to mature before they start laying eggs themselves. This long life cycle makes control easier. Heavy

Fig. 68 Ascaridia, the common large roundworm.

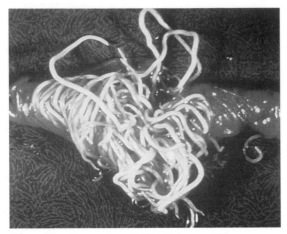

Fig. 69   Intestine full of Ascaridia worms.

infection causes illthrift in the chickens and in laying birds there is often a reduction in the size of the eggs and the shells are whiter than normal. Very occasionally a worm can migrate up the oviduct and get into a developing egg. Infection can also build up in table birds kept on to heavy weight. When the birds are slaughtered the intestines contain large numbers of worms and if they rupture during evisceration this makes the work extremely unpleasant for the poultry staff.

Control

Table birds can be treated with anthelminthic because the withdrawal period for the drug can be completed before the birds are slaughtered for human consumption.

For laying birds the present situation regarding treatment is unsatisfactory because eggs for human consumption have to be withheld from sale for seven days after treatment has been completed. As the course of treatment is for seven days this means that the effective withdrawal period is fourteen days and for many commercial flocks this causes an unacceptable economic loss. The position may change in 1999 because one of the major pharmaceutical companies is hoping to get a zero withdrawal licence for their anthelminthic.

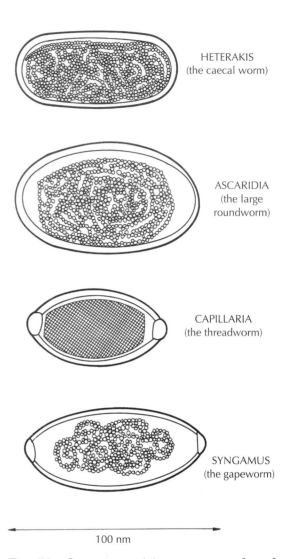

HETERAKIS
(the caecal worm)

ASCARIDIA
(the large roundworm)

CAPILLARIA
(the threadworm)

SYNGAMUS
(the gapeworm)

100 nm

Fig. 70   Some parasitic worm eggs found in droppings.

To get effective control on heavily infected farms a worm dose must be given every two or three months. The programme of control must be linked with hygienic precautions to break the life cycle of the worm and a policy that minimizes the build-up of infection on range areas. The level of infection in a flock can be checked by routine regular examination of droppings and also by post-mortem examination of any birds that die for any reason. A check can be made on the parasites such birds are carrying irrespective of the cause of the death. This is an example of one of the many benefits that can derive from routine post-mortem examinations.

A good egg-producing farmer should aim to manage his flock without the need for drugs after the birds have come into production except in an emergency. Routine dosing during rearing, coupled with hygienic precautions and management calculated to break the life cycle of the worm should be carried out. Technical advice is available for farmers from reputable pharmaceutical companies or their veterinary surgeon.

Caecal Worm (Heterakis)

This is a smaller worm, rather muddy white in colour and approximately 10mm long that lives in the caecum of chickens. It has a short life cycle and only takes 30 days to mature, so control is difficult. It is mainly a parasite of chickens kept on free range. A severe infestation causes debility but it is not a highly pathogenic species. Its main importance is that it acts as an intermediate host for the blackhead organism, Histomonas. Control is best carried out before egg-laying birds come into production or routinely in breeder flocks in which no eggs are sold for human consumption. Control of the parasite in table birds is seldom necessary except on veterinary advice in older flocks if heavy infection has been diagnosed.

Threadworm (Capillaria)

These are very slim worms that are found in the small intestine. Although very small they cause enteritis and illthrift. They can be nearly an inch long but are so fine that they can seldom be seen by the naked eye. Their presence can sometimes be detected by examination of droppings samples but they do not lay large numbers of eggs and infection can easily be missed unless carcasses are available

for a careful post-mortem examination. The worm has a short life cycle and develops in thirty days. Control is as for the caecal worm.

Gapeworm (Syngamus)

This worm lives in the windpipe causing irritation, coughing and respiratory distress in young chickens on range. The worm is red in colour and approximately half an inch long. It is present in pairs in the trachea. Eggs pass out in the droppings. Some are swallowed by earthworms and slugs in which they can remain alive indefinitely. This is the main route for re-infection of chickens and therefore the infection is much more common on old pastures permanently grazed by chickens in which there is a large population of earthworms and slugs. This infection is much more serious in gamebirds than in chickens but can occur on some traditional pure-breed farms. Control must, with this worm, not only be by regular worming of the birds themselves, but by changing the pasture so that the chickens do not pick up new infection from the intermediate hosts.

Tapeworms

These do not cause serious disease in chickens in Britain although they are sometimes present in range birds both during rearing and when adult. The species found in chickens are primarily parasites of wild birds and waterfowl. They all need intermediate hosts to complete their development and are therefore found only on traditional farms where the birds range extensively, particularly onto damp meadows or marshes. Control with a wide-acting anthelminthic is effective.

Coccidiosis

Poultry farmers usually think that coccidiosis is a single disease but there are actually seven quite separate species of

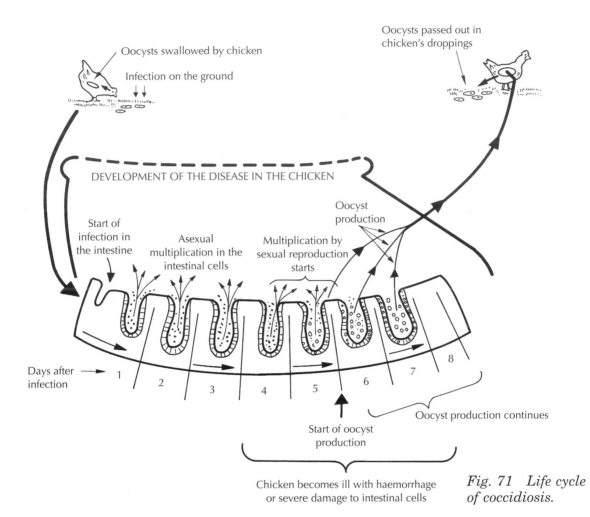

Oocysts swallowed by chicken

Infection on the ground

Oocysts passed out in chicken's droppings

DEVELOPMENT OF THE DISEASE IN THE CHICKEN

Start of infection in the intestine

Asexual multiplication in the intestinal cells

Multiplication by sexual reproduction starts

Oocyst production

Days after infection

1 2 3 4 5 6 7 8

Start of oocyst production

Oocyst production continues

Chicken becomes ill with haemorrhage or severe damage to intestinal cells

Fig. 71 Life cycle of coccidiosis.

coccidia that each cause a different specific disease in chickens.

The coccidial parasites are protozoa, microscopic single-celled animals with a remarkable complex life cycle and an enormous potential for multiplication. One coccidial 'egg' can multiply in a chicken to become over a million new 'eggs' after completing its life cycle that takes only five days.

All the species of coccidia spread from chicken to chicken directly in the same way. Eggs are passed in the droppings and if conditions on the ground or litter are suitable for their development they take less than a week to develop and can then infect a new chicken. They can only develop in moist warm surroundings and are killed by freezing, but if conditions remain favourable for them, as is often the case in British conditions, they can remain alive for over a year and spread the infection from one crop of chickens to another. The outer coat of the coccidiosis egg, the oocyst, cannot be penetrated by most of the disinfectants used in poultry farm hygiene programmes and therefore any remaining in the poultry house can survive after the farm hygiene programme has been completed. This makes coccidiosis particularly difficult to control on broiler or roaster farms.

132

Coccidiosis of one type or another can cause disease from the time the chicks are four days old right up to the time they are in full lay. There are excellent textbooks and illustrated publications that separately describe the different species of coccidia and the particular types of disease that they cause and the interested reader is referred to these. The names of the different species are:

E. tenella, E. acervulina, E. necatrix,
E. brunetti, E. maxima, E. mitis,
E. praecox.

Symptoms

In a serious outbreak affected birds will appear fluffed up and dull and there will also be dead birds present. Often the poultryman will also complain that the litter has gone wet and droppings across the flock as a whole will usually show a marked change from normal. If individual droppings are seen they are likely to be sticky and evil-smelling, darker than normal or tarry and bloody according to the type of coccidiosis in the particular outbreak. In some birds the vent will be caked with abnormal droppings or with white urate material in birds whose kidneys are failing.

A good poultryman should easily be able to recognize a problem in his flock as 'enteritis' when he makes his routine daily inspection of the flock, but the clinical signs of coccidiosis are not completely distinctive and accurate diagnosis will require post-mortem examinations of birds that have died or are showing clinical signs. In less acute cases laboratory examination of droppings can confirm a diagnosis of coccidiosis but the exact species involved will not routinely be established without a complete post-mortem examination.

Almost all chickens pick up a few coccidial parasites under normal poultry farm conditions. For birds going onto

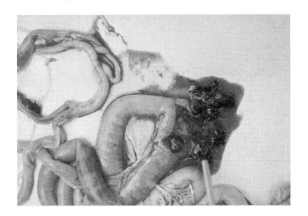

Fig. 72   Intestinal coccidiosis (E. necatrix).

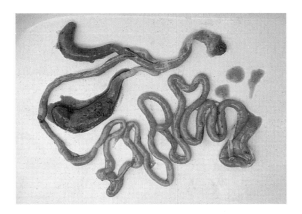

Fig. 73   Caecal coccidiosis (E. tenella).

range and for pullets that are to be kept on as layers, or for any pure breeds, this is essential because the birds only develop an immunity after they have become infected themselves. In a normal healthy flock of chickens the birds will only become ill if they consume a large number of the oocysts at more or less the same time. Good farm hygiene and particularly good litter management and management of areas round feeders and drinkers is an essential protection against the clinical disease because it is in these potentially damp areas that the infection builds up. It is essential for poultry farmers to understand this because the preventive use of anti-coccidial drugs is now prohibited for a number of table bird trademarks, for example organic chicken, and control depends increasingly on good flock management.

Fortunately the ability of birds to develop immunity has made it possible to develop a vaccine. This is effective against all seven types of coccidial parasite and is given during the first fortnight of the chick's life.

Treatment
Treatment of severe infections is necessary as an emergency procedure and will be started as soon as an initial veterinary diagnosis has been made. Continuous preventive medication in the feed is standard practice for table bird production but the medication must be discontinued before the birds are slaughtered so that the necessary withdrawal period required by the medicines legislation is completed before the birds are slaughtered. However, for birds kept on to heavy weight, for those that go out on range and for all chickens that will be reared to maturity it is important that their own immunity to coccidiosis builds up and that they do not remain dependent upon in-feed medication. Needless to say, this immunity can be broken down in birds of any age at any time if their general resistance to disease is lowered. This provides yet another example of how fine tuned is the balance between health and disease in chickens and is another reason why the vaccine has recently been of such benefit to poultry farmers of all kinds.

EXTERNAL PARASITES

Lice

Chicken lice are grey in colour and about 3mm long. They run rapidly over the skin and spend their whole life cycle on the

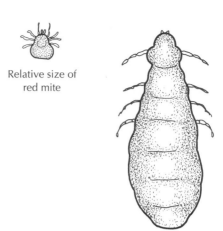

Relative size of red mite

General appearance: Long, yellowish-grey rapidly moving. Legs short and obvious

Fig. 74   The poultry louse.

bird. They lay eggs, nits, on the feather shafts and produce a secretion that sticks the eggs to the feather shaft. Eggs can hatch after about ten days. Lice cause illthrift and irritation to the chickens and severe anaemia in very heavy infestations.

Individual birds can be treated with insecticidal powders or sprays but the louse eggs are protected from the drugs so treatment must always be repeated every ten days until it is established that no unhatched eggs remain and that there are no young lice still on the birds. Antiparasitic powders can also be mixed in with the dust baths in dry weather as an aid in control. If hens that are laying eggs for human consumption have to be treated the choice of drugs that can be used without having to withhold the eggs from sale because of contamination with drug residues is very limited.

Mites

All the species of poultry mite are pinhead in size and can therefore just be seen with the naked eye.

134

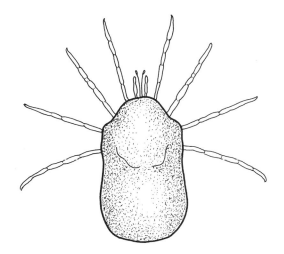

General appearance: Pinhead size. Hard body and distinct legs. Resembles a tiny spider. Moves rapidly

Fig. 75   The poultry red mite.

Red Mite

These mites are reddish-black in colour and suck blood. Infections can rapidly build up in chicken flocks of all kinds and cause severe illness with anaemia and poor production. Affected birds become pale and lose condition, egg production drops and the flock becomes irritable with the result that an outbreak of aggression may occur. Also the poultry staff will pick up the mites which cause severe, although temporary, irritation of the skin and may precipitate eczema in susceptible people.

The mites feed on the chickens at night and spend the rest of their life cycle in cracks and crevices in the poultry house, under crusts of dried droppings and in other suitable places. In a dirty poultry house many can be found in the nesting boxes.

The mites breed in all these locations so that treatment of any that are on the birds needs to be combined with very thorough cleaning and treatment of the poultry house. Treatment is only successful if it follows thorough cleaning of the house so that direct contact is made between the mites and the insecticide.

Regular routine treatments are usually necessary and slats are typical sites where residual infection persists after a single treatment. This is a troublesome parasite to control and repeat treatments are usually necessary.

Medicines legislation prohibits the use of strong persistent drugs during the time a flock of hens is producing eggs, so after an infection has been diagnosed permanent control will depend on breaking the life cycle of the parasites during the time the house is empty or when the hens are not in lay. At this time house maintenance to reduce the number of places where the mites can breed can be carried out and persistent insecticides can be used that have a more permanent effect than those that can be used when birds are in lay. They must however, always be used with great care as they can be toxic to the chickens and easily pollute watercourses where they cause environmental damage.

Northern Mite

This mite is grey in colour. It lives on the chicken for the whole of its life cycle and therefore must be controlled by regular treatment of the birds themselves. In severe infestations this should be carried out every three weeks. Some mites fall onto the litter and into nest boxes so treatment should include thorough disinfection of the house as often as is possible.

Scaly Leg Mite

This mite occurs in pure-breed flocks and in small backyard flocks of chickens. The mite lives under the skin of the leg, causing thickening scaliness and local bacterial infection, but treatment with penetrating ointments containing parasiticide is very successful. Treatment with liquids is ineffective because contact is not obtained between the medicament and the mites, which live quite deeply embedded in the skin protected by the scales.

The Depluming Mite
This species is also occasionally seen. It lives in the feathers and causes local damage to them.

Forage Mites (Fomites)
These are not strictly parasitic but are present in vast numbers in dirty poultry houses, particularly where table birds are grown. They live in the litter and on dead carcasses and cause irritation to birds in a heavily infested house. They can also spread virus infections and should be controlled by a rigorous hygiene programme on the farm. They also cause skin irritation to the poultryman looking after the house.

External parasites are important for four reasons:

- The diseases they cause in their own right.
- They can act as intermediate hosts for other diseases such as cholera and Gumboro disease.
- They cause irritation in the birds and can lead to outbreaks of aggression in infected birds.
- They cause skin irritation to the poultry staff.

New infestations frequently reach a poultry farm in wild birds.

22 The Reproductive System

Egg Production

Wild chickens, like other birds, lay only a fairly limited number of eggs during their breeding season. In some of the pure breeds of domestic fowl high egg production is not an important consideration but in the hybrids developed for commercial egg production selective breeding has dramatically increased the potential number of eggs that can be produced and now over 300 eggs are expected to be laid by each hen during her laying year. Development of this potential for egg production has also taken place in the hybrids that produce broiler chicks. In this case high egg production of the breeder hen is required in order to produce the large numbers of fertilized eggs each day that are required for the commercial broiler market.

Very high egg production puts a severe strain on the hens' reproductive system and makes them very susceptible to reproductive disease problems of all kinds. If a poultry farmer understands the structure and function of the reproductive system he can use this knowledge to keep the birds healthy and producing well. With the assistance of the poultry veterinary surgeon he will be much better able to identify problems and incorporate management factors into his farm programme both to improve the flock's health immediately and also to limit future recurrence of problems that he meets.

STRUCTURE AND FUNCTION

The chicken has only one functional ovary, the right ovary remains vestigeal. The left ovary develops in the midline on the roof of the abdomen just behind the lungs. When it matures it already contains thousands of tiny potential eggs (follicles) and when the bird comes into lay these develop rapidly sequentially and form the yolk of each egg. When active, the ovary overlaps both lungs and kidneys, and the large developing yolks make the organ resemble a bunch of orange grapes of varying sizes.

When a yolk is mature it is budded off from the ovary and, if the reproductive tract is healthy and the bird is not

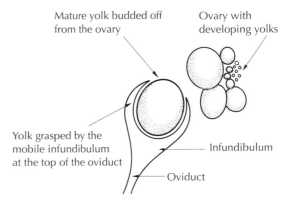

Mature yolk budded off from the ovary

Ovary with developing yolks

Yolk grasped by the mobile infundibulum at the top of the oviduct

Infundibulum

Oviduct

Fig. 76   An egg yolk released by the ovary.

137

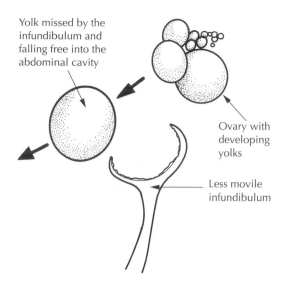

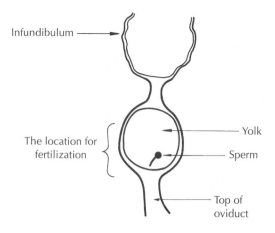

Fig. 78 An egg is fertilized.

Fig. 77 An egg yolk loose in the abdominal cavity.

stressed at this time, it is caught up in the mouth of the wide membranous funnel, the infundibulum, that is the beginning of the oviduct. The infundibulum actively encloses the yolk so that it enters the top of the oviduct and does not fall loosely into the abdominal cavity. The process can be visualized by regarding the infundibulum as a sea anemone grasping its prey.

Yolks that are not successfully grasped fall into the abdomen as 'loose eggs'. If these yolks become infected they cause inflammation and sepsis of the abdominal membranes, 'egg peritonitis', that kills the chicken.

The enclosed yolk then begins to pass down the oviduct and in breeder birds fertilization takes place at this stage. It is therefore essential for the sperm from the cockerel to be able to travel right up the reproductive tract if the yolk is to be fertilized successfully. Clearly, if there is disease of any part of the hen's reproductive tract or if disease in the cock has reduced the viability of the sperm this cannot happen.

The oviduct soon expands into a long thickened glandular tube, the magnum, with a folded spiral lining. As the yolk travels down this tube the white of the egg, the albumen, is secreted round it. If this part of the oviduct is diseased there are abnormalities in the egg white that therefore affect the quality of the egg. The oviduct is commonly attacked by viruses, for example infectious bronchitis virus, and some eggs laid by infected birds will have whites that are watery or have some other defect.

After this long part of the oviduct there is a short length where the shell membrane is secreted and after that the developing egg passes into the shell gland where it remains while the complex shell is deposited on it. Disease, or a mineral deficiency in the hen, can cause malfunction of the shell gland in which case the egg may remain 'soft shelled', or there may be abnormalities in the colour, thickness or texture of the shell. All these are of fundamental importance to egg quality, whether for commercial eggs or the fertile eggs for hatching that are produced by broiler breeder hens.

If the egg is to be laid successfully the vent must also be in good condition. It must be able to dilate to allow the egg to

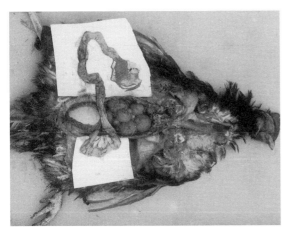

Fig. 79 *Reproductive system of a hen in lay.*

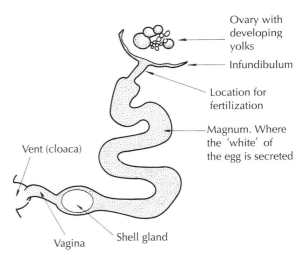

The total length for an adult hen in lay is approximately 24 inches

Fig. 80 *The reproductive system of the hen.*

pass and if this cannot be done the egg will impact in the vagina where it may rupture. Even if it does not rupture immediately it will obstruct the passage of further eggs down the oviduct and these will build up and often become infected, causing impaction of the oviduct and death of the hen.

If the egg cannot be laid without a problem this has an immediate effect back on the ovary and its production of further eggs because the whole complex process of egg production is linked together by hormonal and nervous control.

Growing pullets have to be stimulated to mature and start egg production. In addition to her age and condition, increasing hours of daylight and a rising plane of nutrition contribute to this. A successful farmer must use these factors to programme the development of his birds in order to bring them into lay at exactly the right time so that he has eggs for sale in predictable numbers when he needs them.

Once they are stimulated the ovary and oviduct of a maturing chicken increase in size very quickly and come to occupy a large part of the abdominal cavity. Unless a pullet has a well-developed frame when this happens the space left for the stomach and intestines becomes constricted and

there is less room for food. This very frequently occurs on many poultry farms with the result that the pullets' food consumption actually drops at this time, just when it is essential for it to rise in order to provide enough nutrients both for the beginning of egg production and for the essential continued growth of the pullet.

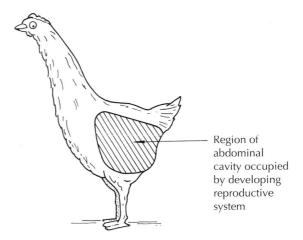

Fig. 81 *In a developing pullet the reproductive system occupies most of the available space.*

A typical brown pullet of a commercial strain should increase in body weight by about 200gm during this period. Failure to achieve this later growth is often the main reason why, on so many farms, the egg production of the young pullets starts normally but then tails off when it is at about 60 per cent.

The birds in flocks with this problem are stressed and very susceptible to disease challenges of all kinds. The flocks do not perform well, there are problems with egg size and quality, mortality in the hens is higher than it should be, and during the second half of their laying life the egg production of the flock falls rapidly. When a pullet comes into lay she suddenly needs extra calcium to form the eggshell. If she has been well reared, has a well-developed bony skeleton and is a good size for her breed she will be able to provide calcium for the first few eggs from her own body reserves but after this she will be dependent on extra calcium, up to a total of 4 per cent in the ration and will also need additional amounts given as soluble calcium grit (often oyster shell). If there is a failure in this calcium exchange the hen will develop brittle bone disease (osteoporosis). This is much more common in flocks of birds kept in cages where it is often coupled with paralysis (caged-layer fatigue). These conditions pose a very serious welfare problem to an affected flock.

The bones of affected hens become severely depleted in calcium, weak and brittle. Affected birds suffer multiple fractures and some become paralysed because of a more severe metabolic calcium deficiency. Affected hens are often crushed by the other birds in a cage.

Birds with fractures should be culled on humane grounds, but some individuals with paralysis will improve if put into a comfortable recovery pen where they have easy access to food and water and are given extra calcium balanced with

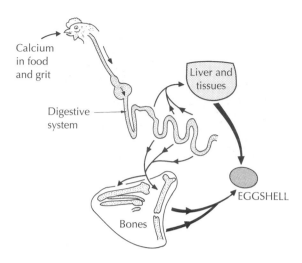

Fig. 82   Calcium exchange in the laying hen.

phosphorus and also additional Vitamin D3. In special cases, emergency veterinary treatment by injection can be successful.

DISEASES OF THE REPRODUCTIVE SYSTEM

These conditions will only be recognized at post-mortem examination, so if they only occur in individual birds in a flock they are unlikely to be spotted. However, if they occur as flock problems a veterinary diagnosis will be made.

Disease of the Ovary

The ovary shows collapsed egg follicles or follicles that have developed on stalks. Diseased yolks are often an abnormal muddy or greenish colour. The cause can be either bacterial or virus infection. Cultures will have to be made to establish the cause. It is very important to establish whether salmonella is present both because of its possible public health importance and the effect on chicks if it is a breeding flock.

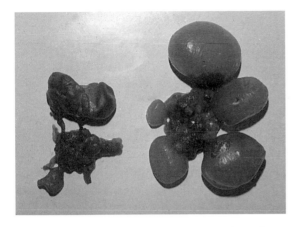

Fig. 83   A diseased ovary with shrunken yolks compared with a normal ovary from a hen in lay.

Egg Peritonitis

The egg yolk fails to be taken up by the infundibulum and falls into the abdominal cavity where it usually becomes infected. The bird's abdomen becomes distended with septic egg material, the abdominal membranes become inflamed and adhesions between the internal organs quickly develop, soon causing death of the hen.

Impaction of the Oviduct

The oviduct becomes blocked with solidified egg material that in most cases is infected. Any yolks subsequently shed by the ovary cannot pass down the oviduct and are therefore voided into the abdominal cavity where they usually become infected and cause egg peritonitis. The affected hen dies from general infection.

Tumours of the Reproductive System

Sometimes the ovary appears grossly abnormal and the bunch of grapes structure is eliminated by a swelling of the whole or part of the organ. The cause is a tumour, often from Mareks disease.

Other types of tumour also occur in poultry and usually affect the membranes supporting the oviduct as well as the ovary.

Diseases of the Vent

● Infection (vent gleet).

Infection is often caused by poor hygiene in the poultry house or from rough protruding fragments of wood, metal, or plastic that irritate or injure the vent when the bird is roosting or laying. Inflammation may also be caused if too much strong disinfectant has been used, particularly phenolic disinfectants or creosote, or by hardwood shavings that have been dressed with chemicals, particularly fungicides. Hardwood shavings are often used in nesting boxes. Any abnormality of the vent causes pecking, both by the bird herself and others that are curious, and haemorrhage commonly results. Irritation is sometimes caused by parasitic infection with lice or mites.

Flock treatment of infections and inflammation of the vent is necessary after the cause is established. Badly affected birds can be treated with antiseptic ointments. Anti-parasitic treatment can be given if necessary and treatment of the flock with antibiotics may be necessary in certain severe cases. Measures to reduce pecking will have to be taken on welfare grounds. These may involve beak trimming and reducing the light intensity. In flocks where only individual birds are affected these should be separated into a hospital pen and individually treated.

● Prolapse.

Straining may cause prolapse, and this may be caused by enteritis, impacted egg material, or inflammation and sepsis of the vent itself.

Congestion of the oviduct can also cause a prolapse. This occurs in young birds in full lay. The prolapse is bright purple in colour and quickly haemorrhages and causes death of the bird. Peck wounds usually increase the amount of bleeding. This type of prolapse sometimes occurs as a serious flock problem in birds that are brought into lay too quickly. This causes excessive congestion of the blood vessels in the whole of the reproductive tract. In severely affected flocks radical treatment is sometimes necessary to reduce egg production. This can be achieved by reducing the number of hours of daylight and reducing the quality of the food. To avoid the problem developing in subsequent flocks the birds must be brought into lay when they are older or more gradually.

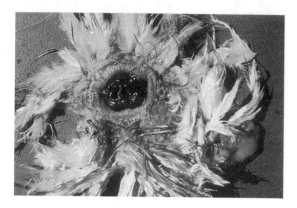

Fig. 84   Prolapse of the vent.

REPRODUCTIVE PROBLEMS IN THE COCKEREL

Poor fertility may be the result of very poor nutrition and condition, abnormal development of the testes, or infectious disease. Abnormalities of the vent must always be considered when investigating an infertility problem. Inflammation, sepsis or caking with faeces or urate material is easily seen and individual treatment may be carried out by the poultryman. If it is thought that a cockerel is infertile a test can be carried out on his semen either by natural mating or using artificial insemination techniques. Microscopic examination of the semen for sperm numbers and characteristics is coupled with cultures to identify any bacterial infection. A blood test will also be carried out. Mycoplasma is the commonest infection to cause infertility and the infection can be spread to the hens at attempted matings. Tumours of the testes caused by Mareks disease are common in heavily infected flocks.

Poor libido leads to absence of successful mating and will clearly result in infertility in flocks where only one cock is available. Poor libido may be the result of poor nutrition, parasitic infection or disease. It is often temporary in immature cockerels that have been reared in the absence of pullets. These birds take time to settle down and are often initially bullied by the females. In flocks with several cockerels present the more submissive birds are often bullied by the other cockerels. These birds become severely stressed, lose condition and may die from kidney failure.

23 Failures in Egg Production —

The success of both commercial egg producers and poultry-breeding farms of all kinds depends on the number and quality of the eggs laid by the individual chickens. A pure-breed farmer needs healthy chicks to maintain and develop his blood lines, for show and for sale. A commercial breeding farm needs healthy hatching eggs for sale and a commercial egg farm, whether large or small, needs hens to produce predictable numbers of eggs of consistently good quality. Any failure in egg production will quickly turn a profitable flock into one that loses money. Often this is not only because of a fall in egg numbers but because there is an associated drop in egg quality. This leads to dissatisfied customers for eggs taking their business elsewhere and to poor hatchability in breeding flocks.

Disease challenges to laying birds do not always show up as obvious illness and deaths but almost all of them quickly have some effect on egg production and with some diseases these effects can be disastrous. Very often the effect on egg production is the only obvious sign that a poultryman sees at the beginning of a disease outbreak. There may not even be a very significant change in the food and water consumption of the flock. All poultry farmers need to identify the reason for any failure in egg production as soon as possible and it is useful to put the different types of failure into categories and relate these to their most likely possible causes.

Complete Failure of Egg Production

● Failure of pullets to grow to adequate weight.
Due to poor rearing. Poor nutrition and heavy parasitic infections may be contributory factors.

● Incorrect lighting pattern during rearing.
Pullets kept on natural management systems that begin to mature towards the end of the summer are affected by the shortening hours of natural daylight in the autumn between August and December. If these birds are not given supplementary light during this time they often do not come into lay until the following spring when the days get longer again and the intensity of the light increases.

● Pullets become too fat.
If the maturation of the pullets, particularly the heavy pure breeds, broiler breeders and some egg-producing hybrids that tend to put on weight, is delayed they will lay down so much free fat that the further development of their reproductive system is inhibited, even when external conditions are correct. Reasons for failure to mature include feeding a ration with too high an energy value but very low in protein, such as when supplemented with ad-lib whole grain or maize, and shortening hours of daylight during the autumn

and winter. Birds of this kind will often not even come into lay in the spring and if they do start to lay, their production will be poor and there will probably be deaths from fatty degeneration of the liver.

● Developmental failures.
Individual birds will fail to develop, as in all species. Chicks that have certain types of infectious bronchitis early in their development may have reproductive failure as a result. The virus attacks the immature oviduct and prevents further development. Early vaccination of pullets prevents this problem and it has been rare in recent years. The ovaries of these birds develop normally but the eggs are shed into the abdomen and subsequent death from egg peritonitis is common.

● Tumours, circulatory disease or serious infections of any kind in individual birds. These will clearly prevent egg production.

● Very acute severe disease in the flock. Usually this will cause a reduction rather than a complete cessation of egg production in a flock but occasionally very virulent Newcastle disease, influenza, cholera or egg drop syndrome will cause a complete cessation of egg production.

Poor production in the Flock from the Start of Lay

● Poor development of pullets, poor nutrition, incorrect lighting pattern, poor management.
Clearly the reasons are the same as those in flocks where there is no egg production at all.

● Infections in the pullets during growth that have become chronic.
Parasitic infections and mycoplasma are typical examples.

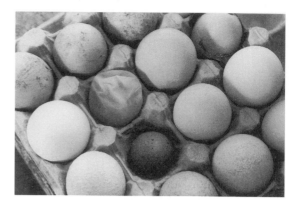

Fig. 85 Second quality eggs (dirty, double yolker, small, stippled shell, thin shell, soft shell, pale colour).

Drops in Egg Production in Flocks That Start Normally

In the many cases where there is no obvious illness in the birds the quality of the eggs that are laid often gives clues to the cause of the problem. If the cause is a nutritional, management, or stress factor a good poultry farmer will be able to recognize it. In all other cases and where there are no clear effects on individual egg quality a detailed veterinary investigation will have to be made.

● Eggs pale in colour.
The sudden appearance of a significant percentage of pale or chalky white eggs usually indicates infection. However, it is sometimes seen in free-range flocks when no cause can be found and in these cases the eggs usually return spontaneously to normal after a few days.

● Eggs mottled in colour.
This is most often seen in young flocks. It is thought to be stress-related but the cause can often not be found and the condition is only temporary.

● Eggs small.

This may indicate parasitic infection or a nutritional fault. It also occurs in pullets that are brought into lay too young with too low a body weight.

● Double-yolked eggs.

A small number of double-yolked eggs are acceptable in a flock but if a large number occur it usually indicates stress during the time the birds are actually laying an egg. There is a close link between the moment when the hen lays the egg and the time that the next egg to be laid leaves the ovary. If there is interference with this complex mechanism, for example if the hen is frightened when she is on the nest or there is excessive competition with other hens at that time, the ovary may subsequently release two eggs simultaneously and these will be enclosed in a single shell to produce a double-yolked egg.

● Absence of the shell (a soft-shelled egg)

Some young pullets coming into lay produce several soft-shelled eggs before they come into lay properly. This is an adolescent fault and is temporary. Soft-shelled eggs in birds of any other age are usually a prelude to a significant reduction in egg numbers in a flock that has contracted a severe infection. Viruses are often responsible, for example egg drop syndrome, infectious bronchitis and Newcastle disease. Very severe lack of calcium available for the hens will also cause soft shells but this does not usually happen suddenly (see below).

● Eggs with thin shells.

This may be a sign that the hens are receiving a ration significantly short of calcium, in which case it may be associated with brittle bones (osteoporosis) and possibly paralysis in some of the hens if they are kept in cages. Often, however, the condition is caused by infection in the hens, usually with viruses.

● Eggs with abnormal shells.

The shells may be porous or have a rough sandpaper texture. They may be pale and chalky, have irregular thickness or have distinct lines and grooves in the shell. There may be line cracks.

All these abnormalities are very often an indication of virus infection. The viruses destroy some of the cells in the shell gland of the bird so that the shell is not laid down evenly. The viruses most commonly involved are the various types of infectious bronchitis and egg drop syndrome.

● Eggs of abnormal shape.

This is frequently stress-related, a disturbance to the hen's behaviour leading to retention of an egg in the shell gland. Double-yolked eggs are extreme examples. Like most shell abnormalities it can also be the result of virus disease.

● Eggshell blood-stained.

This occurs in pullets that have come into lay too quickly with congestion of the reproductive tract. In this case, it is often associated with a high incidence of prolapse in the flock. It also occurs sometimes after a change of feed.

● Eggs stained with droppings.

Eggs with poor quality shells pick up faeces so dirty eggs may be associated with any of the conditions described above. Enteritis in the hens is indicated if there are no other abnormalities in the eggs.

● Abnormal yolk.

If yolks are very pale the cause may be lack of pigment-producing substances in the birds' food, for example xanthophyll and carotene. Artificial pigments are now banned from incorporation into poultry foods under food legislation. Pale yolks often indicate a parasitic infection in the birds. Other cases occur, particularly in free-range flocks, where the cause cannot

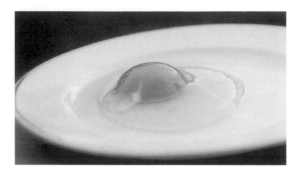

Fig. 86a   A good egg with a firm compact white.

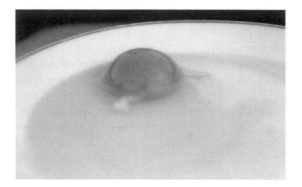

Fig. 86b   An egg with a watery white spreading over the whole plate.

be identified and the colour returns to normal after a few days.

● Abnormal whites.

The white of the egg (albumen) is produced in the oviduct. Abnormality indicates disease in the oviduct. The whites of affected eggs are watery. When eggs with this abnormality are cracked into a pan the white spreads out over the whole pan. The cause is usually virus infection of the cells in the oviduct that produce the albumen. The fault is often permanent in flocks that have suffered from infectious bronchitis, Newcastle disease or egg drop syndrome and is economically disastrous for the poultry farm because it leads to customer complaints. When a normal egg is cracked there is a dense portion of the white which remains close to the yolk and increases the height of the egg. This height can be measured and is an indication of the quality of an egg. The measurement is in haugh units. In badly affected eggs the yolk membrane is also affected and the yolk also spreads.

● Blood spots and brown 'meat' spots in eggs.

These can indicate disease or over-activity of the oviduct in birds at peak production. In small flocks their presence can often be traced to individual hens and

can be attributed to slight faults in their individual reproductive systems.

Inability of the Hen to Lay the Egg

This is a problem frequently identified by owners of small backyard flocks, pure-breed flocks or pet hens. In commercial flocks affected hens that are found by the poultryman are more usually culled. Causes can include:

● The egg is too large, probably a double yolker.
● The egg has a rough shell that lacks lubrication.
● The egg has broken internally.
● Immaturity in pullets with very small frames.
● Disturbance during laying leading to impaction of the egg.
● Disease of the vent.
● Disease in the hen causing her to be unable to strain to lay the egg. The cause may be distension of the abdomen from circulatory disease and dropsy or tumours.

Infected eggs

Eggs, whether from commercial flocks for human consumption or from breeder flocks, can carry infections. These can spread from one generation of chickens to the next and, in some infections, cause human food poisoning.

The most important of these organisms are salmonellae, mycoplasma and some viruses capable of transmitting diseases such as infectious runting and stunting and viral arthritis that are of commercial importance in broilers and roasters.

In flocks heavily infected with large roundworms a worm can occasionally get into the oviduct and become enclosed in an egg. These eggs are clearly disastrous to the reputation of the producer and although they do not occur often they are a strong reason for regular routine worming of all flocks before the birds come into lay and good hygiene to control any build-up of worms in the environment for flocks.

Infertile eggs in Breeder Flocks

Infertile eggs are those that do not start development and must not be confused with eggs that start to develop but fail to hatch. The causes of infertility often relate to the cockerels and the management of the breeding flock. Failure of eggs to hatch may be the result of infection in the eggs themselves or infection picked up in the hatchery or under the broody hen. In any flock, fertility should be over 90 per cent and hatchability over 75 per cent and if these levels are not achieved the reason for the failure should be established.

Later History of a Flock That Has Had an Egg Production Problem

When the possible causes of a problem have been considered, confirmation by specific blood tests and probably post-mortems on birds that are typical of the condition may be necessary. From the results of these investigations the vet will be able to give an informed opinion on the future performance of the flock. After

some problems production may be expected to return to normal quickly but in others, particularly those that are the result of virus or mycoplasma infections, erratic production and a persistently higher than normal percentage of second quality eggs are likely to persist and the birds may go out of lay at a much younger age than in a healthy flock.

TREATMENT OF INDIVIDUAL BIRDS

Whole impacted eggs can sometimes be removed by gently infusing liquid paraffin or an alternative emollient lubricant round them through the cloaca and then by careful manipulation. Surgical removal is not usually satisfactory because the vent is damaged and the passage of further eggs is made impossible.

Broken eggs can less often be satisfactorily removed because of the difficulty

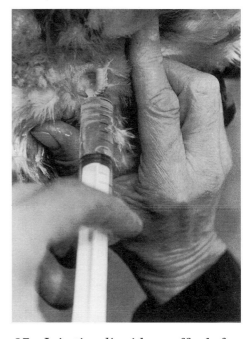

Fig. 87 Injecting liquid paraffin before removal of an impacted egg.

of removing all the shell fragments. Repeatedly flushing the cloaca and vagina with lubricant can be helpful. Antibiotic treatment should be given to the hen to combat infection of the reproductive tract and antiseptic ointment should be applied to the vent.

Infections and Injury to the Vent

The first priority for the poultryman is to establish the reason for the damaged vent as it may indicate a flock problem not confined to an individual bird. Individual birds may be treated with antiseptic ointment. Aerosol sprays should be avoided because they dry up the vent and make the passage of subsequent eggs impossible. In any case some degree of fibrosis of the vent usually occurs and makes it impossible to return affected birds to the main flock because subsequent eggs produced will impact. In flocks where vent gleet (infection of the vent) is widespread, antibiotic treatment of the flock may be necessary.

24 Diseases in Day-old Chicks ——

The signs of ill health in baby chicks are described in detail in Chs. 5 and 6.

A good poultryman will spot that there is something wrong with a batch of chicks very quickly, but it will often not be obvious how the problem arose. He should record how the illness first showed and the age of the chicks when the problem first appeared. After that a picture of the problem can be built up and an accurate diagnosis usually made, with the assistance of the vet if necessary. It is important that the progress of each flock is recorded accurately in case a problem has to be referred back to the suppliers of the chicks or of the food for possible compensation. If this is the case it is essential that the vet is involved so that his report can be added in support of any claim that has to be made for compensation.

The pattern of a specific disease outbreak will usually be able to be identified roughly within one of the following categories:

- Mortality starting at the hatchery immediately after the chicks hatch.
- Mortality or illness occurring during the first twenty-four hours after the chicks reach the farm.
- Mortality and illness persisting after the first three days.
- Mortality and illthrift starting at about the third day and persisting into the second week of life.
- Mortality rising during the second week of life.

- Illthrift and unevenness without significant mortality developing from five days old and being quite obvious by the time the flock is two weeks old.

Many small-scale poultry keepers breed their own replacement chickens. Failure of their eggs to hatch, or the presence of disease in the baby chicks that do hatch is a common disaster for many of them and these problems should be investigated immediately with their vet. The problems that they experience on a small scale are the same as those that determine the success or failure of a commercial hatchery and its reputation for selling healthy day-old chicks to their customers.

Baby chicks can become ill for a number of different reasons:

- They can be carrying infections transferred to them in the egg from the parent breeder. The chick's development starts as soon as a fertile egg is incubated. The twenty-one days between that and the time it hatches can be compared to the period of pregnancy for a calf or any other mammal.
- They can pick up infection at the hatchery or in transit to the farm.
- Development in the hatchery depends on the correct conditions of incubation and the absence of any infections picked up there either before or after hatching. They can pick up infections from the broody hen in both the above ways.

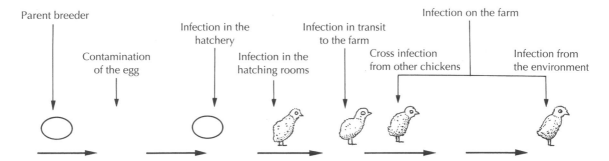

Fig. 88 The ways in which eggs and baby chicks can become infected.

- They can pick up infections on the poultry farm after they are housed.
- They can become ill because of faults in the environment in the hatchery, in transit, or on the farm.
- Chicks hatched under a broody hen can pick up infection at any stage of their development according to the health status of the parent breeder and the broody hen, and the hygiene of the broody coop or shed.

DISEASES THAT MAY BE TRANSFERRED FROM THE PARENT BREEDER

These diseases are very easily missed by both the poultry farmer and the vet because they can show in such a variety of ways. There may be a failure of the eggs to hatch, chicks may be weak at hatching and show disease and high mortality during the first few days, or they may start to grow normally and then show characteristic disease symptoms later on. Some chicks may never show clinical signs at all but remain as dangerous symptomless carriers for their whole life and others only show signs of disease if they suffer from some stress or pick up another infection that acts as a trigger for the latent infection.

All poultry farmers must realize however, that most of these egg-transmitted infections can also be picked up by the chicks after they hatch, either from a contaminated environment on the farm or by cross infection from other infected birds.

Infections that can be passed on from parent breeders include:

Salmonella Pullorum (BWD)

Causes early diarrhoea and mortality.

Salmonella Enteritidis

This is of particular importance because infection can also be passed to people and cause salmonella food poisoning. In chicks the disease can cause high early mortality, diarrhoea and degeneration of the hip joint.

Salmonella Typhimurium

Unfortunately it has recently become established that chicks can occasionally become infected with *Salmonella typhimurium* via the egg.

Epidemic Tremor (Avian Encephalomyelitis)

Causes muscular tremors, convulsions and other severe nervous symptoms in

150

chicks, usually starting after the chicks are a week old.

Chick Anaemia Virus

Causes illthrift and anaemia, and an affected flock becomes very variable in size and condition after they are two weeks old. Affected birds are more susceptible to other diseases.

Mycoplasmal Infections

These cause very poor hatchability because some of the developing embryos are killed by the bacteria. In chicks that do hatch there are seldom any respiratory signs at first, but chicks may be unthrifty and have higher than normal mortality. Birds carrying infection are more susceptible to other respiratory diseases and to E. coli, and if any other disease occurs it is more severe than in an uninfected flock. In older birds mycoplasma on its own shows as respiratory disease or lameness, according to the type of mycoplasma present.

Leucosis Virus (Big Liver Disease)

This cancer, common in some pure breeds, spreads from generation to generation.

Runting and Stunting Viruses

It is now established that some of the viruses that cause malabsorption can be egg-transmitted. However, newly hatched chicks also pick up these infections very quickly after hatching, either at the hatchery or on the farm. They cause enteritis and illthrift.

Nutritional Deficiencies

Although these are not infections poultry farmers must remember that the development of the chick before it hatches is

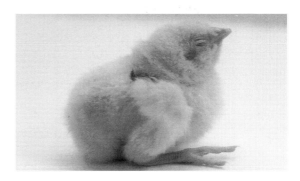

Fig. 89 A chick unable to stand.

dependent on the quality of the egg and this is affected by the quality of the ration given to the breeder hen. Nutritional deficiencies can show as failure of eggs to hatch, weak chicks, or chicks that hatch with clearly identifiable abnormalities. These include gross deformities, abnormal feathers, curled toes, inability to stand or nervous signs. Some of these conditions are easily confused with early infection in the chicks.

Control

If an egg-transmitted infection is suspected it is most important that the breeder flock is identified so that the birds that are carrying the infection can be treated or culled. They are the primary source of the infection. Infected chicks can sometimes be successfully treated, but treatment is never simple and must be carried out systematically under the direction of the vet.

In pure-breed flocks, or chicks from small breeders or collections, the identity of the affected parent breeders can be established fairly readily with the full cooperation of the farmer. Although it is disappointing for a breeder to discover that he has carrier birds in his flock, action must be taken to eliminate these egg-transmitted infections from their flocks if he is to succeed.

If the chicks came from a commercial company the company should always be informed. Clearly it is in the interests of any successful company to identify problems in their birds so that action can be taken.

DISEASES THAT CAN BE PICKED UP BY THE CHICKS BEFORE THEY ARE DELIVERED

These conditions are easier to recognize because the chicks show clinical signs within the first few days of life.

● Infection from Dirty Eggs Set.
When the hygiene control at the hatchery is poor or if dirty eggs are set infections can penetrate through the shell of the eggs and infect the developing chicks. Some of these eggs will not hatch and if broken open will be found to be foul-smelling and to have green or brown evil-smelling yolk. Some of the chicks that do hatch are also likely to be infected and will quickly spread infection to other chicks in the same hatching tray or chick box before delivery to the farm. Chicks, like mammals, have a navel cord along which nutrients are absorbed while they are still in the egg. The navel is still wet when the chicks hatch and bacteria, often E. coli, salmonellae or streptococci, can infect newly hatched chicks through their navels. The organisms then quickly multiply in the yolk sac. The infection very often generalizes and mortality is high.

This type of infection can become established in the setter machines, the hatcher machines, and also in the chick sorting rooms at hatcheries. If a large number of the chicks have picked up infection of this kind an observant poultryman may notice that the flock has an unpleasant musty smell. He may also notice that some chicks have tense swollen abdomens and protruding navels. Post-mortem examination of chicks that die shows gross infection of the yolk sacs and general infection in many of the chicks. The carcasses of affected birds rapidly decompose after death.

If only a few individual chicks are infected the affected chicks will die during the first three days of life and then the mortality will drop to almost zero. If, on the other hand, cross-infection between chicks has occurred the mortality will rise again after the third day as newly affected chicks start to die. This mortality will then persist well into the second week of life unless urgent action is taken and antibiotic given to the flock. The chicks that pick up the infection later on will not have yolk sac infection because the navels dry up during the first thirty-six hours after hatching and the yolk sacs are resorbed and disappear. The later affected chicks will have general bacterial infection that will be detected at post-mortem examination.

● Aspergillosis.
The fungus Aspergillus fumigatus can become established in a hatchery and can infect the developing eggs. Most of the infected eggs will not hatch, some will be 'bangers' and spread infection within the incubator. Live chicks that do hatch will pick up fungus spores in the hatchery and quickly develop pneumonia. This is called brooder pneumonia. After delivery to the farm the poultryman will notice that some of the chicks are breathing more rapidly than normal, sometimes with their beaks open. Many of the chicks die quickly and those that are affected but have not died remain unthrifty and very susceptible to other diseases because Aspergillus is one of the infections that interferes with the development of the bird's immune system.

This fungus disease is fairly common in pure-breed farms and on small farms where eggs are incubated by traditional methods. On these farms the fungus multiplies in damp straw or musty hay that is used as bedding or in nesting boxes, and in stacks of spoiled straw or hay bales on the farm.

● Spraddle Legs and Inability to Stand.
Sometimes chicks arrive on the farm unable to stand or with legs widely apart. The cause may be that they have been on a slippery surface when they have hatched or that they have been put on to a slippery surface in the sorting room at the hatchery. In other cases it is because the quality of the air in the hatcher machines was poor and the chicks were not able to expand their lungs fully during the first few minutes after hatching. Occasionally the cause is poisonous fumes such as excess formaldehyde or other disinfectant in the hatchers. In these cases post-mortem will show that the lungs have not expanded fully in addition to dislocation of the hip joint. If problems of this type occur they should always be referred back to the hatchery.

● Chick Nephropathy.
In some flocks there is very high mortality from kidney failure during the first three days of the chick's life. This condition is easily diagnosed by post-mortem examination. Kidneys are grossly abnormal and often urate has accumulated in the tissues. The chicks are dehydrated. Careful investigation often reveals an environmental fault in the hatchery although in other cases no obvious cause can be established and it has been suggested that a very early virus infection can sometimes be responsible.

● Runting and Stunting.
These viruses can be picked up at the hatchery if the sorting room or vehicles used for transporting the baby chicks are infected.

● Poor Quality Chicks.
The chicks will be of uneven size and the level of activity will be poor. Some will fail to find water and food and mortality will be high during the first twenty-four hours. Mortality will persist at an unacceptable level in chicks that fail to start to grow, 'non-starters', and die as starve-outs up to the time they are about nine days old. There will be wide variation in size and development of the chicks that survive.

DISEASES ARISING ON THE FARM

Disease conditions are likely to show as illness and mortality in the chicks that persist beyond the third day. Causes include:

Poor Early Environment, Management and Nutrition

Management of baby chicks has been described in Chapter 3. Signs of a serious fault will include chicks that are slow to start, respiratory failure, variable development and a high percentage of starve-outs right up to the ninth day.

Infection in the House Prepared for the Chicks

The cause is a poor hygiene programme or reinfection of the house during the farm clean down. Common infections are E. coli, salmonella, runting and stunting viruses, Gumboro disease, staphylococci. On small traditional farms aspergillus infection may be present in brooders that have not been fully disinfected.

Infection from Other Birds on the Farm

From droppings, in the air, or on the poultryman's clothes and boots.

Infection from the General Farm Environment

Infections of this type are very commonly seen in practice. The usual reason is that areas outside the individual poultry houses have not been included in the clean-down programme. Resistant bacteria, viruses, and infections that spread via intermediate hosts and vermin can all persist in the environment for long periods (see Ch. 28).

New Infection Reaching the Farm

New infection may be introduced to the chicks in wind currents or from passing transport, feed lorries or visitors to the farm. The poultryman can also introduce additional infections if he has a new flock to look after. Salmonella may also occasionally be present in starter feed. This is now rare in Britain.

25 Vaccination

Vaccines are given to enable the chickens to resist specific infections. They act by stimulating the immune system, unlike antibiotic 'medicines' that act directly on the organisms that cause disease.

When a vaccine is given it stimulates cells in the immune tissue to produce chemical antibody that can then counteract a future infection. Others, memory cells, store knowledge of the disease. If these cells recognize the infection again at any future time they instruct the antibody cells to manufacture additional antibody very quickly to boost the immune response of the bird to the disease.

Two types of vaccine have been developed:

Dead Vaccines

Extracts are made from cultures of the disease organism that have been killed in the laboratory to make them harmless. The extracts are still capable of stimulating the immune system if they are injected into a bird. In most killed vaccines a single dose does not stimulate enough immunity for the bird to resist infection completely and a second dose after an interval of two to four weeks is necessary.

Live Vaccines

There are two types of live vaccine used in poultry.

1. A naturally occurring organism closely related to the one that actually causes the disease, but that cannot cause clinical symptoms, is grown by the pharmaceutical company in the laboratory. Because it is related to the disease organism it is able to stimulate the chicken's immune system.
2. The actual disease organism is modified in the laboratory so that it is no longer capable of producing serious disease but retains its ability to stimulate immunity.

ADMINISTRATION OF LIVE VACCINES

Some live vaccines have to be given by injection, for example Mareks disease.

Some have to be given individually to the chicken. Infectious laryngo tracheitis vaccine has to be administered by carefully dropping a dose of vaccine into the eye and

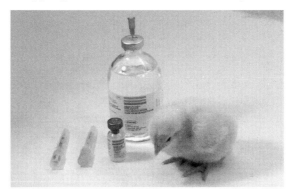

Fig. 90   Equipment for vaccination against Mareks disease on a small farm.

155

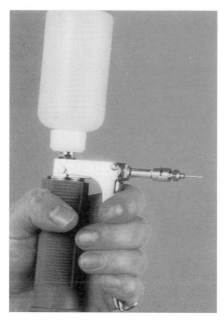

Fig. 91   A Kaycee multidose syringe.

Fowl pox vaccine has to be given by scarifying the skin.

Other live vaccines can be given by mass medication. Vaccine for all the birds in a poultry house is mixed with their drinking water so that they all drink a sufficient amount of the vaccine water to stimulate an immunity. An alternative method suitable for some vaccines is by administration of an aerosol spray. Here the vaccine is mixed with water and the solution is sprayed onto the birds. Immunity is produced by the vaccine contacting the eyes of the chicken, or being swallowed.

Some live vaccines, for example the 'strong' Gumboro disease vaccine and the vaccine against coccidiosis, only need one dose to be effective but for most of them two or more doses are needed. The live vaccines against infectious bronchitis and Newcastle disease cannot on their own produce an adequate immunity to last for the whole life of a layer or breeder flock and for chickens of this type they must be supplemented with a dose of dead vaccine

which is given by injection just before the birds come into lay.

It seems like stating the obvious to emphasize that it is useless for a poultry farmer to give vaccines to the chickens at all unless they *work*! However, in poultry veterinary practice countless disease problems occur in flocks in which vaccination has been carried out but has not produced a satisfactory immunity so that the flock later suffers clinical disease from a condition against which it was believed to be fully protected.

Vaccination, whether of a child against measles, a puppy against distemper or a chicken against infectious bronchitis, is a very delicate biological procedure. Like all biological procedures it can never be 100 per cent effective and the effect depends greatly on the ability of every individual chicken to respond to vaccination. Every poultry farmer can, however, make certain that the factors over which he has control are always carefully checked and that the method and timing of vaccinations is correct. Vaccination is a skilled operation and shortcuts must not be taken. Full use should always be made of the technical back-up services provided by all the good pharmaceutical companies that manufacture vaccines, and every vaccination procedure should be carried out strictly according to the method recommended. Vaccination programmes should be designed for their flocks, whether large or small, with the assistance of the vet and the vaccine manufacturer. Periodic checks should also be made to ensure that their vaccination procedures are effective. Unless this is done farmers often have a sense of false security. Checks are usually made by blood tests carried out under the supervision of the vet.

When a chicken receives a live vaccine the organisms in the vaccine multiply in the chicken and give it a mild attack of the disease. This is what is commonly called the vaccine reaction and unless it occurs the vaccination is ineffective. During the time that a bird is suffering from this vaccine reaction it is very susceptible to other diseases and it needs special care over this period.

If a chicken gets too many different vaccines over a short period of time its immune system becomes overloaded and it will fail to respond fully to any of the vaccines given.

The principle of vaccination is to *prevent* disease, in contrast to medicines that *treat* disease organisms present in the bird. It follows that birds must be vaccinated *before* they meet the field infection. This is why the timing of all the vaccines in each poultry flock is so important and why a vaccination programme must be carefully worked out for a specific farm.

Live vaccines are very fragile and the living organisms in them quickly die. If they have died the vaccine is useless and cannot stimulate any immunity. When they are administered in water, live vaccines are quickly killed by:

- Chlorine present in the water.
- Other disinfectant or detergents in the water.
- Algae, sediment or rust in the water.
- Being delayed in the pipework between the insertion point and where the water is drunk by the birds. For this reason it is usually unsatisfactory to administer vaccine through the header tank in a poultry house.
- Residual disinfectant in the drinkers.
- Delay by the poultry vaccination team between reconstituting the vaccine and administering it to the birds in the correct amount.
- Failure of birds to drink adequate vaccine within the short period before the vaccine dies.

When administration is by aerosol they are ineffective when:

- Droplets in the spray are the wrong size.
- Contact between the droplets and the beak and eyes of the birds being vaccinated is not made.
- The environment of the house where the vaccination is being done destroys the vaccine. This will happen if the humidity is too low.

Before a vaccination using live vaccine is carried out the poultryman should go through a simple check list. This should include:

- Vaccine must be within the stated expiry date.
- Vaccine must have been stored continuously at the correct temperature.
- Vaccine has not been overheated or suffered excessive changes in temperature before being reconstituted.
- Water used for reconstituting vaccine contains no chlorine. For water administration adding skim milk at the rate of one pint per two gallons improves the viability of the vaccine.
- Drinkers and equipment must have been thoroughly cleaned with water and not disinfectant or detergent.
- The method of distributing vaccine between the birds must ensure that they all receive vaccine before it dies. The maximum time that a vaccine is viable after reconstitution, even under correct conditions, is:
  - for respiratory vaccines – 2 hours
  - for Mareks vaccine – 4 hours
  - for Gumboro vaccine – 8 hours.

The amount of water needed to dilute the vaccine clearly depends on the method used to distribute it between the chickens, the age of bird and their water consumption, and the number of birds in the house. Detailed recommendations on how to calculate the correct amount are always given with recognized vaccines and can be

Some Vaccines That Are Used for Chickens

Dead vaccines given by injection:

Organism	Comments
Pasturella	against cholera
Newcastle disease	
Egg Drop Syndrome	
Gumboro disease	for breeder birds to give immunity to their chicks
Salmonella enteritidis	there is no vaccine against other salmonellae

Live vaccines:

Method	Examples and Comments
Given by injection	Mareks disease
Given by eyedrop	Infectious laryngotracheitis
Given by skin scarification	Fowl pox
Given by aerosol	Some respiratory virus vaccines
Given in drinking water	Infectious bronchitis There are several strains of this virus disease, but vaccine is only available against some of them Newcastle disease Coccidiosis Gives protection against all the seven types of coccidia found in chickens. Care must be taken that no in-feed anti-coccidial drug is present in the feed at any time either before or after a flock is vaccinated

discussed with the supplier or the vet. The birds must be thirsty when the vaccine is administered and water must be withheld for a time before a vaccine is given. The best time of day for vaccination, the simultaneous availability of food for the birds and the length of time that water should have been withheld are all important considerations but generalization on an exact method suitable for all flocks is not possible.

ADMINISTRATION OF DEAD VACCINES

Dead vaccines must be administered accurately so that each bird receives an effective dose. With multidose syringes for administration it is essential that there are no air bubbles or airlocks in the apparatus.

The operation must always be carried out methodically and there must be enough members of a vaccination team to ensure everyone's safety. Some dead vaccines are very dangerous if injected by accident into poultry staff when they are vaccinating chickens. If this does happen the farm's doctor must be notified immediately and the patient should go without delay to the casualty department of the local hospital, taking details of the vaccine from one of the bottles in use. Speed is essential, as a severe skin reaction develops very quickly.

26   Treatment ————————————

It is easy to forget that the very first antibiotic drugs that could kill specific disease organisms were only developed in the 1930s. There were no specific drugs at all that were effective against septic wounds in the 1914–18 Great War but sulphonamides were used with success in the Spanish Civil War. It was not until 1950 that penicillin began to become widely available in human and veterinary medicine. Since then a wide variety of drugs have been developed and used in humans and in animals, including poultry, and people have come to think of antibiotics as the only effective treatment for disease.

Recently, governments have begun to encourage a shift away from the general use of antibiotics in animals that produce food for human consumption like chickens, and increasingly tough legislation now progressively limits antibiotic use to specific circumstances. There are two main reasons for this:

- The first is to try to reduce the incidence of resistance to antibiotics that has developed in certain strains of bacteria that can cause disease both in man and animals.
- The second is a part of the general effort by governments to reduce contamination of food products with additives. This is a factor in their strategy to reduce the increasing number of people who suffer from allergic diseases.

The ways of treating disease in chickens can be considered within three main categories:

Drugs that Kill the Organisms That Cause Disease

- Antibiotics.
- Anticoccidials.
- Anthelminthics.
- Parasiticides.

Specific medicines should always only be used after an accurate diagnosis and under the direction of the vet. The forward policy for repeat treatments is often an important part of the successful control of a disease on a farm and this will frequently be combined with recommendations on vaccinations and farm hygiene.

Viruses are not killed by antibiotics but the severity of virus diseases, for example infectious bronchitis and runting and stunting, is often increased by secondary bacterial infections. When antibiotics are properly used they can often help to control these, shorten the course of the disease and hasten recovery in a flock.

Whenever drugs are given the farmer must keep complete records of their use and must ensure that the statutory withdrawal periods are completed after a course of treatment before the poultry or eggs are sold for human consumption. Care must also be taken that drugs cannot spread in water or food to other batches of chickens or other animals on the farm.

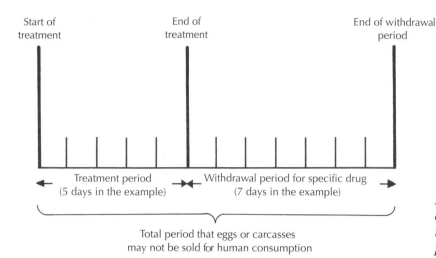

Start of treatment

End of treatment

End of withdrawal period

Treatment period
(5 days in the example)

Withdrawal period for specific drug
(7 days in the example)

Total period that eggs or carcasses
may not be sold for human consumption

Fig. 92   Treatment with antibiotics. Calculating total withdrawal periods.

Dosing

Correct dosing with drugs is essential for successful treatment. A large number of farmers do not appreciate this simple fact and inadequate or irregular dosing of chicken flocks is one of the main reasons for failure of a disease-control programme.

If a person with a severe headache needs two aspirins to control the pain there is little point in him just taking half of a single aspirin! If he dissolves the two aspirins in a full glass of water he must drink *all* the water in order to consume the full dose of aspirin.

Exactly the same logic relates to dosing a chicken. If the bird weighs 1kg and needs 1gm of antibiotic each day to control a disease it must get the full dose if the drug is to be successful. The 1gm dose can clearly be administered individually by injection, or it can be mixed with a small amount of water and given directly into the beak. Individual dosing is, however, impossible for large numbers of chickens and usually the drug is best given dissolved in the day's drinking water for the whole flock. It must be mixed with the amount of water that the birds will actually drink, even if they are sick, over a 24-hour period if the individual birds are to get enough drug to be effective.

If farmers remember this simple principle of treatment they can work out ways of dosing the birds that will be successful with the help of the vet. Some useful points to remember are:

- Do not mix medicine with more water than the birds will drink over the calculated period.
- Make up medicines fresh each day if possible.
- When dosing through a header tank tie up the ball valve, otherwise the medicine will progressively dilute with water and birds will not get an accurate dose.
- Allow for reduced water consumption of birds that are sick.
- Allow for any reduction due to the palatability of the medicated water. Some drugs have a bitter taste. Ask the vet whether to add glucose, vitamins or some other substance as a palatizer.
- Make certain that there are plenty of drinkers in order to encourage maximum water consumption by the birds.
- Use only high-quality medicines and check the solubility before starting dosing.
- Clean the water system, pipework and so on with a water sanitizer after a course of treatment. This will stop

160

water blockages occurring from the build-up of algae in the pipes. Some medicines encourage algal growth. Cleaning water pipes by using a sanitizer should be a part of routine management. If pipes block up it takes a busy poultryman several hours to clear them and during this time an emergency water supply must be made available for the birds.

Methods That Act by Blocking the Effect of Disease-Producing Organisms

Competitive Exclusion

A competitive exclusion product consists of a preparation of live, useful bacteria that are normal inhabitants of the intestines of healthy chickens. In the chicken the purpose of these bacteria is to help them to maintain a healthy digestive system. The best commercial competitive exclusion products consist of a mixture of over sixty kinds of these useful bacteria. They are dried into a powder like instant coffee and can be resuspended in water and administered to the chickens either as a single dose in their drinking water or as a spray.

Competitive exclusion products are proving to be increasingly valuable aids in the control of bacterial diseases in chickens, particularly salmonella. The principle is to give chicks a full dose of these useful bacteria as soon after they hatch as possible. When they are swallowed and reach the intestine the bacteria start to multiply and very soon line the intestine, providing a protective coat that prevents harmful bacteria that the chick may swallow later on from finding room to become established, multiply and cause disease.

One of the weaknesses of modern systems of poultry management is that, to eliminate the disease organisms in the chickens' environment that can persist from one crop of birds to another it is necessary to carry out a very thorough disinfection between each crop of chickens that are reared. Unfortunately normal bacteria are also killed by the disinfection programme and this means that the baby chicks do not pick up as many useful bacteria during their first few days of life as chickens that are reared traditionally. This leaves them much more susceptible to the bacteria that can cause disease, such as Salmonella. Competitive exclusion treatment gives the chicks the normal useful bacteria that they would acquire naturally in the wild, without the risk of harmful bacteria that could cause disease being included.

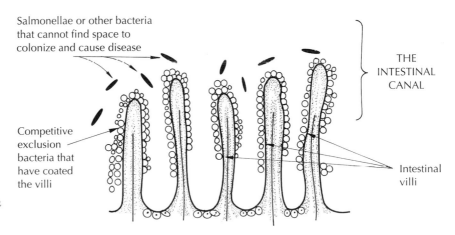

Salmonellae or other bacteria that cannot find space to colonize and cause disease

THE INTESTINAL CANAL

Competitive exclusion bacteria that have coated the villi

Intestinal villi

Fig. 93 How competitive exclusion works.

A competitive exclusion product can also be given to chickens at any age in order to re-establish their normal digestive bacteria after a course of antibiotic has been given.

Probiotics
Probiotics are also suspensions of useful bacteria. The difference from competitive exclusion products is that they do not contain as many species of bacteria and those present do not necessarily become permanently established in the intestine. They are therefore given more continuously to chickens in order to assist in maintaining a healthy intestine and also to increase the bird's resistance to disease. Both types of product can be used as aids in maintaining what can be described as 'positive health' in a flock. However, care must be taken only to use products that are manufactured by recognized pharmaceutical companies as there are a number of inferior products on the market.

Changes in Nutrition
Some infections are more likely to occur in chickens that are fed on particular types of ration. This is also the case with sheep, pigs and other domestic animals. A change in nutrition may be advised by the vet as an integral part of the treatment for some specific diseases.

Additional Treatments to Improve the Health of the Birds

Since antibiotics have been used on a large scale many poultry farmers have come to rely on them completely for the treatment of disease, and accessory treatments to hasten recovery or build up the resistance of a flock to infections has been neglected. The importance of the poultryman himself has been diminished and this has been a very real weakness in the management of poultry farms. The effects that additional methods of treatment, when coupled with good husbandry, can often have on the success of the disease-control policy on a farm cannot be overemphasized. Management tools that the good poultryman can use as aids in health control include:

- Improving the environment for the chickens, for example by temperature control and litter management.
- Changing the food to give a convalescent diet with increased digestibility. This may have an altered protein and energy specification and will probably have a higher overall vitamin content than a standard ration.
- Administration of electrolyte solutions in order to increase water consumption and improve kidney function.
- In severe illness giving glucose in the drinking water in order to provide instant energy. This is of great value in young chicks. As with any medication, care is needed because an excessive amount may cause diarrhoea.
- Giving water-soluble vitamins in therapeutic amounts to improve digestion and impaired metabolic processes.
- Booster vaccinations.
- The use of probiotics or competitive exclusion products.

27 Handling and Treating Chickens ─────────────

Catching Individual Birds

Catching a small number of birds is, if possible, best done during hours of darkness when the birds are sleeping. The birds can then be caught individually without disturbing other birds in the flock. A bird should either be caught by putting both hands over its back firmly, pressing the wings into the body to prevent flapping, or alternatively by grasping both legs firmly at the hock. For examination, an individual bird should then be brought into an upright position against the catcher's body, restraining the wings with the spare hand. Take special care if the

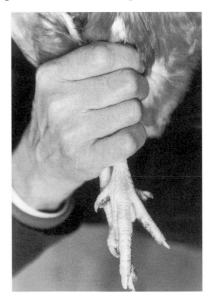

Fig. 94 Catching a chicken. Both hocks must be grasped tightly.

bird has spurs, they can be very sharp and cause a nasty injury to the catcher.

If a bird is caught correctly it is seldom very stressed and further procedures can usually be carried out easily.

Handling Small Groups of Birds

The birds should be gathered into a corner of the building using a high wire screen and caught individually when they are cornered. They will be less stressed if they have the minimum amount of room from which to attempt to escape.

Catching Chickens for a Blood Test

If the testing is to be carried out away from the poultry house one or two spare empty crates will be needed. Catch up the required number of birds, put them into crates and transfer them to the place where the operation is to be carried out. After each bird has been sampled put it into one of the spare crates, otherwise it will prove virtually impossible to identify which birds have been tested and much time and patience will be wasted. This very often happens in practice!

Blood Sampling

The blood will often be taken by the vet or by a qualified technician, but the poultryman can make the job much easier if he handles correctly the birds that are presented for testing.

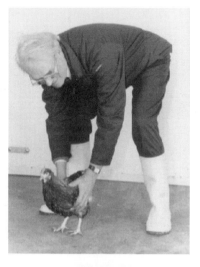

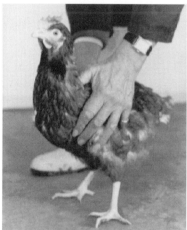

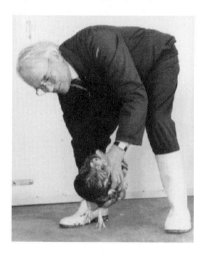

Fig. 95   Picking up a chicken.

Blood sampling should be done using the wing vein, the ulnar. The operation is much easier if the birds are restrained in a fairly natural upright position. Most birds remain quite unstressed in this position. The catcher must first grasp both hocks firmly and then hold the bird against his body in an upright position. He should then grasp both wings at the elbow joints and bring them together above the bird's body. The wings must be held firmly enough to immobilize them but not so tightly that the return of venous blood in the wing vein is impeded. This often happens when the handler is too tense and lacks confidence. The legs of the bird should be held slightly away from the handler's body so that the wing with the exposed vein presents an oblique surface for the blood tester. This makes penetration of the vein with the needle much easier.

The bird can easily be reversed to present the other vein for the blood tester if required.

Blood testing

Equipment needed
- For most chickens over twelve weeks old a needle 0.8mm × 16mm (21 gauge × 5/8) is satisfactory, used with a plastic 2–3ml syringe.
- Prepare an adequate supply of clean water for rinsing syringes and needles, and a bowl or bucket for discarded water.
- Prepare a rack containing the required number of blood sample bottles of the size and pattern requested by the testing laboratory. Have a few spare bottles handy.

Technique
- Gently adjust the position of the chicken's wing so that the vein is fairly engorged.
- Align the needle and the vein carefully.

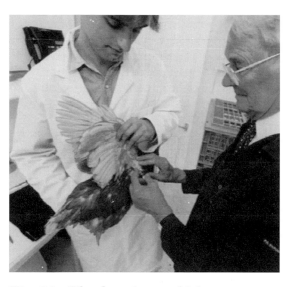

Fig. 96 *Blood-testing a chicken.*

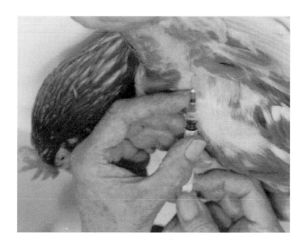

Fig. 97 *Blood-testing a chicken, close up detail of injection.*

- Push the needle into the lumen of the vein with a single firm movement, and then along the vein for a short distance. The needle must be sharp.
- Gently withdraw blood into the syringe. Do not hurry. 1.5–2ml is adequate for most tests.
- Remove the syringe from the vein.
- Check and release the chicken. A small amount of haemorrhage from the vein is acceptable.
- Without delay, or the blood will clot, gently squirt the blood into one of the previously prepared blood sample bottles. Do not squirt it in too quickly, this will damage the blood and reduce the accuracy of the test.
- Immediately rinse the syringe and needle several times in clean water before the blood clots. Discard the rinsings. Needles and syringes can be re-used until they become contaminated with blood or until the needle becomes blunt.
- The blood samples taken should then be handled strictly according to the instructions of the laboratory. If they are not handled properly the blood will

not clot satisfactorily and will not give accurate test results, making the whole operation worthless.

If the vein is incorrectly punctured and blood will not flow into the syringe it may be possible to catch sufficient blood to perform some of the tests from the slight haemorrhage from the damaged vein that usually occurs. A blood sample bottle is wiped against the vein to catch the drops. Clearly, blood collected in this way is of inferior quality and the sampling procedure is less humane for the chicken.

Blood sampling is a very skilled procedure and a poultryman who needs to learn the technique will require personal training and plenty of practice before he becomes competent.

Injecting Chickens

Needles must be clean to avoid spread of infections between chickens.

- When injecting live vaccines, for example Mareks disease, needles cannot be disinfected using disinfectant because this kills the vaccine. Needles should therefore always be changed as often as possible during vaccination of a flock to reduce the possibility of cross-infection on a dirty needle.

- When injecting dead vaccine or therapeutic drugs, disinfection of the needles can be carried out during the work run. Several needles should be in use simultaneously and the spare ones should be kept in a saucer of methylated spirit. The needles can then be used sequentially and replaced into the spirit when they are changed. This ensures that cross-contamination on dirty needles is limited and reduces the possibility of the septic injection abscesses that are a common and unwelcome sequel to injections that have been carried out without adequate hygienic precautions being taken.

Site of Injection
- When injections are made into the neck it is important to avoid injecting into the fibrous tissue. Care must be taken to get the injection into the loose region just under the skin. Also it is impor-

tant to avoid injecting too near to the back of the bird's head. If an injection reaction develops there the bird will be unable to bend its neck to feed or drink.
- Injections into breast muscle should be avoided wherever possible in chickens that are being reared for meat production. The site of the injection can remain as a blemish in the breast meat.
- When injecting into a leg, care is needed to avoid the hock joint region. Also an injection must not be made near to a bone. The reaction will cause severe lameness.

Dosing Chickens

Individual dosing of chickens with a syringe is very successful if it is carried out correctly. The most difficult problem is usually for the vet, who has to calculate doses for individual chickens instead of being able to mass medicate a number of gallons of water for a whole flock!

The bird to be dosed should be unstressed. Chickens panic if they are placed on a slippery surface and dosing must be carried out in a suitable location. The

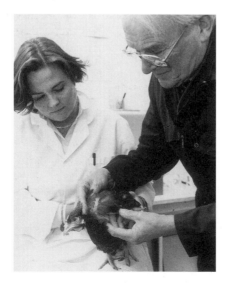

Fig. 98a   Injecting a chicken into the neck.

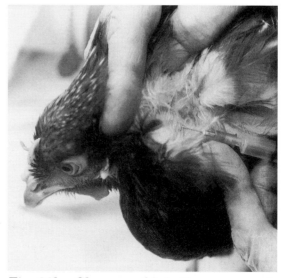

Fig. 98b   Close-up of injection.

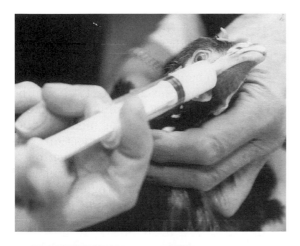

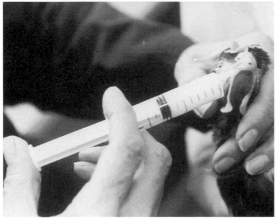

Fig. 99 Dosing individual chickens requires patience and can be messy.

assistant should restrain the bird in as natural a position as possible, keeping one hand over the tail region or round the wings to prevent the bird backing away from the person administering the dose, and pressing the bird down fairly firmly. The administrator should then gently manipulate the neck until the beak is directed upwards. The beak can then be opened using the plastic nozzle of the syringe and the dose slowly and steadily trickled in. Some may be dribbled out and lost and it is wise to allow for this by putting a 25 per cent coverage of the calculated dose into the syringe.

Peck Wounds and Aggression

The injured birds and, if possible the bully birds, should be removed from the flock. Peck wounds are best treated with a purple antibiotic aerosol spray advised by the vet. This controls haemorrhage and dries up the wound. In most, but not all, chickens the purple colour does not excite the curiosity of other birds so further pecking does not occur.

Fractures and paralysis

Severely injured birds should always be placed in a warm comfortable hospital pen or box where they cannot further damage themselves before they have been examined fully by the vet. First-aid treatment for a bird with a fractured or paralysed wing can be to strap the wing close to the body in as natural a position as possible using wide sticky tape which is wound right round the body of the chicken.

Crusted Eyelids and Conjunctivitis

Antiseptic or antibiotic ointment advised by the vet should be rubbed into the affected area generously once or twice a day to break down the scabs and allow the eyes to open fully.

Distended Sinuses

The vet may suggest attempting to clear these as part of more general treatment. If the nostrils are blocked with exudate they should be bathed with warm water and cotton wool and then an attempt made to express the distended sinuses through the nostrils by squeezing sinuses in an upward and forward direction.

Impacted Eggs

The technique for dealing with this problem is described in Ch. 22.

Overgrown Beak and Nails

These can be trimmed using a sharp pair of nail clippers or secateurs. A clean cut should be made and care taken not to trim down to the sensitive vascular tissue and cause haemorrhage.

Beak Trimming

Routine beak trimming of chicks at the hatchery is now being discontinued. Beak trimming is classed as a mutilation and should only be done for specific flocks on advice from the veterinary surgeon.

In addition to preventing aggressive behaviour it restricts the ability of the birds to pick up food, to preen and to drink. The vascular tissue at the base of the beak is very sensitive and inflammation and infection commonly follow beak trimming. The procedure should only be carried out on welfare grounds to prevent aggression in specific flocks.

If required, beak trimming may be carried out during the first 72 hours of the chick's life using an approved machine, providing the operation is under the permanent supervision of a trained operator. After this age, beak trimming must only be done under direct veterinary supervision.

Only the upper beak must be trimmed and less than one-third should be removed. Trimming must under no circumstances be so severe as to expose the nasal passages and any bleeding should be minimal. A straight cut can be made across the upper beak but it is less inhumane to limit the cutting to rounding off the upper beak so that the birds cannot grip with it and inflict serious damage to other birds by aggressive behaviour.

Beak trimming can be carried out on any age of bird, including adults. The operation is best carried out using very sharp secateurs. A clean cut causes less tissue damage than cautery.

A suitable food that the birds can easily pick up should be given for a few days after trimming and a vitamin tonic is often beneficial.

28 Disease Control by Hygiene

In order to design an effective hygiene policy for disease control on the farm every poultry farmer should have a working knowledge of:

- The ways in which infections can spread from chicken to chicken.
- How the various disease organisms can remain alive on the farm and the length of time that they can survive before they are picked up by another chicken.
- The correct way to use disinfectants.

Chickens of any type that are healthy are much better able to resist infections than those with an underlying infection such as Gumboro disease, those that are stressed because of bad management on the farm, or those under conditions of extreme intensification. If a flock is to remain healthy it must be in balance with its environment and a good poultry manager will aim to keep the level of exposure of the flock to disease organisms under control. The aim must be to keep the levels of all infections as low as possible, to build up the natural resistance of the birds by good management practices and to supplement this with the use of vaccines, competitive exclusion products and preventive medication when necessary. Poultry farms that are haphazardly run on extensive lines almost always have a consistent disease problem that they never completely overcome.

Even on farms where only one age of bird is kept and there are no remaining chickens on it when the between-flocks cleaning schedule is carried out, it is not possible to completely eliminate every disease-producing organism from the farm. However well-maintained the poultry house is there will be cracks and crevices where dust containing bacteria and viruses can persist, and often where mites and litter beetles can remain alive under the insulation of the building. Also the areas outside the individual poultry houses can harbour infections such as runting and stunting viruses and Gumboro disease that will recontaminate the house even before the next batch of chickens arrive. These basic problems are, of course, even more difficult to control on multi-age farms, where birds have access to free range, on pure-breed farms or collections open to the public, and on traditional back-yard flocks.

Hygiene control on all farms will include:

- An effective Everyday Hygiene Programme.
- A rigorous clean-down schedule after each house is empty.
- A programme for disease control of all the areas outside the individual poultry houses, including the paddocks on free-range farms.

Every control policy should have four basic aims:

- To limit as much as possible the number of new infections that can reach

169

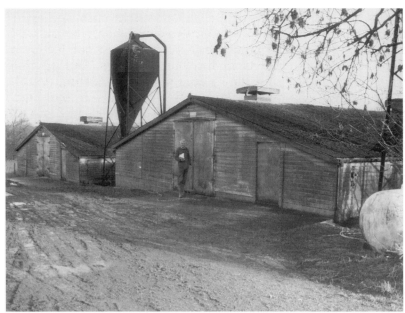

Fig. 100 The clean-down is a difficult job in wet weather.

the farm. This is what is meant by Unit Security.

- To keep the level of all infections on the farm as low as possible with an effective everyday hygiene programme.
- To remove or kill with disinfectants the maximum number of infectious organisms when each poultry house becomes empty by designing a between-flocks sanitization programme.
- To ensure that the hygiene measures taken on the farm include control of infections that are present *outside* the individual poultry houses, and also parasites and other organisms that can become established in the grazing paddocks.

Disinfectants

MAFF publish a list of Approved Disinfectants that have been tested to give satisfactory control of specific infections if they are used correctly. Disinfectants are usually inactivated by dirt and organic matter of all kinds, direct contact must be made between the disinfectant and the infectious agents if the organism is to be killed. In practice this usually means that

it is better to incorporate a detergent (a foaming agent) into the disinfectant so that dirt can be effectively removed during disinfection.

Many poultry farmers falsely believe that a disinfectant will kill all the organisms that cause disease under any circumstances. This is quite wrong and they must be used correctly according to the manufacturer's instructions just the same as antibiotics and vaccines if they are to be effective. A normal cleaning programme will therefore comprise firstly, the removal of all gross dirt and secondly, disinfection, which itself may have to be carried out in two stages. On large poultry farms a final stage of Fogging is often carried out, so that disinfectant in the 'fog' penetrates fan shafts, ducts and other areas inaccessible to the standard cleaning programme.

Unit Security

The possible introduction of new infection onto a poultry farm or into a poultry house should always be considered by the poultry farmer.

170

● Visitors.

Visitors should be checked and should always wear protective clothing. Contract workers for catching or vaccinating birds are particularly likely to bring infection onto the farm. The managing director and the vet should also comply with the disease precautions laid down! On farm shops customers should be kept as far away from the actual chickens as possible and the risk of infection from visitors to collections and exhibitions of poultry that are open to the public should always be kept under review.

● Transport.

Feed lorries and any vehicles that have visited other poultry farms always present a potential risk, particularly of course if it is known that there is a serious epidemic of any particular poultry disease in the area. In these cases all visitors or vehicles arriving at the farm should be reduced to the absolute minimum.

● Wild Birds.

It must be accepted that wild birds are a threat to flocks of chickens. Diseases that can be introduced include mites, roundworms, cholera, salmonella, Newcastle disease and avian influenza.

It is good policy to use wire netting to prevent access to buildings by wild birds and to limit cross-contamination on range as much as possible. Practical ways of achieving this will vary from farm to farm.

● Vermin.

Rats, mice, other mammals, flies, mites and beetles can all introduce new infections onto a farm. They can also maintain the infections once they are introduced by acting as intermediate hosts for the disease organism or parasite. A continuous policy for the control of vermin of all kinds should be a part of normal farm management for all efficient poultry farmers.

● New Chickens Brought onto a Farm.

Newly brought-in birds should be isolated as much as possible from other birds on the farm for fourteen days. During this time any necessary blood testing, vaccination, preventive medication and anti-parasitic treatment can be carried out.

● Airborne Infections.

Epidemic diseases can be brought onto a new farm in wind currents. Virulent forms of Newcastle disease, avian influenza and infectious bronchitis can all be introduced in this way. There is little that the poultry farmer can do about this on established poultry farms but if sites for new houses are being considered, prevailing wind, airflow, and the location of existing farms should all be considered before deciding where to put up a new building.

Effective Everyday Hygiene Programmes

● Drinkers should be cleaned daily. Scrubbing with an iodine disinfectant that includes a detergent is ideal. Iodine is particularly good for controlling algae and slime and is not very corrosive. It also has a low toxicity for the chickens, the detergent makes cleaning easier and the poultryman can see that he has carried out the job effectively because of the brown colour of the disinfectant. In practice this is a very important point to consider.

● Feeders should be kept physically clean and disinfected as often as practicable. Birds must not be able to walk in or roost on feeders.

● Any dead birds must be collected and disposed of quickly and efficiently. Carcasses must be bagged or burnt and must not be contaminated by flies which will reintroduce infection into the house. The incinerator should be placed well away from all the poultry houses to avoid cross-contamination

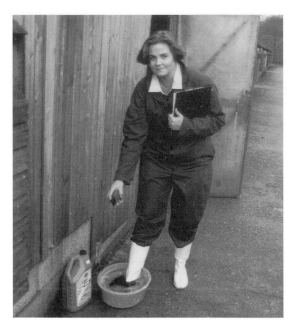

Fig. 101   Disinfection. Footbath and protective clothing.

with feathers and ash. This is another common cause for the spread of infection back into buildings on farms.

- A footbath containing fresh disinfectant at an effective strength should be maintained outside each poultry house. This both reduces spread of infections from droppings on the poultry staff's shoes or boots and more importantly, serves as a constant reminder to everyone on the farm that hygiene is important.
- All staff should wear protective clothing that is only used on the poultry farm. Protective clothing should also be available for visitors to the farm. The clothing should be washed or changed regularly.

BETWEEN-FLOCKS SANITIZATION PROGRAMMES

A standard programme will include:

- Removal of gross dirt.

- Cleaning and Disinfection of the House. Poultry farmers can obtain comprehensive advice on individual sanitization programmes from the technical staff employed by good disinfectant manufacturing companies or from the vet. The quality of disinfectants available varies greatly and they should never be purchased purely on a least-cost basis. Lots of water is the best least-cost disinfectant; a fact that many farmers do not recognize!

- Application of a Long-Acting Insecticide.
This is wise in order to reduce the build-up of mite infections and therefore to control infections for which mites and other parasites act as intermediate hosts.

- Checking Effectiveness of the Programme.
After cleaning has been completed areas can be tested by swab testing to check the numbers and types of bacteria still present. Swabs can be taken under the supervision of the vet and the swabs will be examined by a microbiological laboratory. Results must be clearly interpreted if they are to be of value to the farm, and should always be recorded for future reference.

The Areas Outside the Poultry Houses

On many farms the cleaning programme does not include these areas adequately and often houses actually become reinfected from the surrounding areas during the cleaning programme if this is carried out badly. Important points that must be considered include:

- Vegetation between the houses must be well managed.
  Large amounts of dust are produced continuously in any poultry house and this dust contains any infectious organisms that are present in the house. It settles better in vegetation than on concrete or asphalt but must not be allowed to build up, so the vegetation must be well-managed.
- No spare equipment or rubbish should be stacked close to any of the poultry houses. This collects dust and attracts vermin.
- Tractors, trailers and farm machinery used during the clean-down can reintroduce infection into the houses that have already been cleaned. Cross-contamination from this source should always be considered and vehicles should not be parked overnight near to the poultry houses that have already been cleaned.
- Droppings, litter and other bedding.
  This must be carted at least 200yd away from the buildings and stacked or spread so that reinfection in wind-blown dust or by flies does not occur. Dust must not blow back from trailers and so forth into houses that have already been cleaned.

Straw bales, hay and so on should be properly stored. Any musty materials stored in the open near to poultry houses will introduce fungus infection into the house and will also harbour vermin.

- Maintenance of the building.
  It is important to repair defects in which infections and vermin can remain at this time.

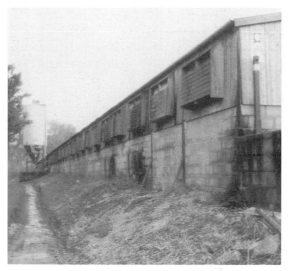

Fig. 102
Vegetation must be managed to make vermin control possible.

- A rigorously applied vermin control programme for the farm.

Problem areas that often contribute to the failure of the sanitization programme include:

- Electric fittings.
  These cannot be wetted and are often therefore not included in the sanitization programme.
- Water system.
  Complete sanitization of all the pipework and drinkers must be carried out to prevent the slow build-up of algae in the system. This is a common cause both for blockages of the water system and difficulties in carrying out water medication effectively on farms. Regular sanitization of water pipework should also be included in routine farm management.
- Header tanks.
  These must be kept with well-fitted lids, otherwise dust constantly falls into them and continuously reinfects birds with bacteria and viruses that are present in the house.

- Food preparation areas.
  These are often omitted from the sanitization programme and become heavily contaminated with dust that can contain disease organisms.
- Poultry staff canteens, office, toilets, and so on.
  These are also often omitted from the clean-down and can maintain infections on the farm between flocks.
- Ceiling areas, insulation, fan shafts, air inlets.
  These are difficult to reach. Removal of dust with an industrial vacuum cleaner and a final fogging are sometimes advisable.
- Earth-floored buildings.
  These should be generously sprayed with a recommended heavy-duty disinfectant after litter has been removed and cleaning completed. This will reduce the carry-over of infection with coccidia and worms in addition to bacterial and viral infections.

SPECIAL POINTS FOR FREE-RANGE AND PURE-BREED FARMS

- Moveable houses and runs.
  Pure-breed farms and the smaller egg-producing farms on which birds are housed in moveable coops are ideally suited to implement a really effective programme for disease control. Coops can be dismantled and disinfected regularly and then moved onto clean ground so that parasitic and other infections including coccidiosis do not build up on the farm. This is an excellent system if well managed.
- Rotational grazing
  Paddocks for grazing should be used sequentially and managed to reduce the carry-over of parasitic infections between flocks. Ploughing and reseeding, leaving fallow, and grazing with sheep can all be usefully incorporated into the regime.
- Protection from wild birds
  If the chickens are fed outside, for example to encourage them to use the whole of their range area, contamination of the feeders by wild birds is likely. Feeders should be covered in order to limit this and the poultryman should be aware of the potential disadvantages of this practice.

INDEX